With love and admiration to my mother, who taught me to think for myself and to cherish children

To parents who have children with hemophilia: You are so lucky! This child of yours will open up new worlds for you, take you places you never dreamed of, and teach you a new language of medical terms. You will get to meet wonderful people you never would have met. You will discover strengths that you didn't know you possessed and find out that you can fight tooth and nail for the child of your heart. Ultimately, you will be transformed into a better, more caring individual who savors life each day.

–Dorcas Walker, author, mother of a child with hemophilia

Contents

Foreword vii
Points to Remember ix
Introduction xi
1   "Your child has hemophilia." 1
2   What Is Hemophilia? 17
3   The First Few Months 37
4   The Doctor-Parent Partnership 57
5   The First Year 75
6   Becoming a Savvy Consumer 91
7   Prophylax—and Relax! 113
8   Fostering Healthy Self-Esteem 131
9   Hemophilia at Home and on the Road 151
10 School Days 167
11 Sports and Summer Camp 183
12 Family Matters 197
13 Deciding to Have More Children 213
14 When an Inhibitor Strikes 229
15 Understanding Your Insurance Coverage 245
16 Maintaining Your Insurance Coverage 265
17 Adolescence and Beyond 273
Conclusion 289
Notes 293
Acknowledgments 301
Appendices 305
   A. Publications and Resources 305
   B. Pharmaceutical and Medical Device Companies 317
   C. Sample Letters 319
   D. History and Significance of Blood Product Safety 324
   E. Medicines to Avoid 334
   F. Factor VIII Dosage Calculation Chart 336
   G. Product Trademarks 338
Glossary 339
Index 361

Foreword

Twenty-five years ago, the Internet was a fledgling experiment. Social media simply did not exist. And the term *virtual communities* could only have been uttered in one of the *Star Wars* movies. In short, information and engagement were not as readily available as today. At that time, people diagnosed with hemophilia and their families had limited sources of information about this rare bleeding disorder. And the parents of hemophilia patients often struggled to find needed emotional and educational support.

Fortunately, Laureen Kelley recognized the challenges facing the bleeding community as the mother of a child with hemophilia, and did what she does best: took action. Laurie possessed the foresight, energy, and courage to research, write, and launch *Raising a Child with Hemophilia: A Practical Guide for Parents*, providing a breakthrough guide for parents of children diagnosed with hemophilia. She based the book on her personal experiences managing her son's bleeding disorder, and she tirelessly gathered insights and knowledge from over 160 other families. Finally, hemophilia families had an insightful resource to help them cope with their children's disorder.

In this fifth edition, *Raising a Child with Hemophilia* has never been more relevant, especially in today's complex healthcare environment. Through her writing, Laurie has initiated a new genre: parents of children with hemophilia now have a voice, they are empowered, and they are actively engaged on important topics with caregivers, policymakers, and other stakeholders. In this latest edition, Laurie has provided incredibly practical guidance and knowledge spanning a quarter century. Her book continues to serve as a unique, stellar reference for hemophilia patients and their families.

As a groundbreaking author and active champion for the hemophilia community, Laurie's work has impacted thousands of lives worldwide. Most significantly, she has served as an inspiration, sending the strong and meaningful message that children with hemophilia and their families are not alone on their journey. Like Laurie, CSL Behring understands the unique challenges faced by hemophilia patients and their families. We have been pleased to support Laurie's efforts over the years because CSL Behring works every day, around the world, to provide solutions to the same challenges. *Raising a Child with Hemophilia* has provided educational and emotional support for more than a quarter-century to a community at the heart of our work, and will continue to do so in this revised edition. We are pleased to champion this type of patient-centric program that so perfectly complements the work we do.

Thank you, Laurie, for your unyielding and energetic leadership on behalf of the hemophilia community. You have made a lasting difference in our world!

Paul Perreault
CEO & Managing Director
CSL Limited

Points to Remember

Although mainly boys get hemophilia, some girls do have hemophilia. For the sake of simplicity, in this book we'll refer to a child with hemophilia as "he."

In the first four editions of this book, we included quotations from over 100 parents. When *Raising a Child with Hemophilia* was first published in 1991, the Internet was in its infancy. There was no Google, no Facebook, no texting. *Raising a Child* was the go-to source to read about other parents' experiences with hemophilia and learn firsthand what to expect. From the mid-1990s through the mid-2000s, families with hemophilia communicated with each other through the Internet using text-only mailing lists and bulletin boards. The early 2000s saw the introduction of the first social media sites, and since the birth of Facebook in 2006, social media has exploded. In this fifth edition of *Raising a Child with Hemophilia*, we've removed most of the parent quotations. All the medical, treatment, and parenting information here has been researched, checked, double-checked, and reviewed by medical staff. The content was and still is determined by what parents tell us is important for other parents to know.

Glossary terms are in light bold at first appearance. Note that some glossary terms appear for the first time within a bolded heading.

Although this book has been extensively researched, no book is a substitute for medical care with a hematologist at a hemophilia treatment center (HTC). Always call your HTC for medical advice concerning hemophilia.

Introduction

Hemophilia: It's Not What You Think

On a brilliant, frosty day in New Hampshire, a 10-year-old boy straps on a snowboard and joins his classmates entering the lift line. He's an excellent student and has also taken snowboarding lessons for several years. As the lift nears the top of the mountain, he prepares to glide onto the intermediate trail that he wants to master.

In a dojo at a karate school in Kansas, a thirteen-year-old boy prepares to take his black-belt exam. After seven years of lessons, he can break boards with his feet and topple a larger opponent. He's slim and wiry, with well-developed muscles. His joints are in excellent condition. Above all, he has sharp mental concentration. His *sensei* smiles as this young student enters, bows, and begins his exam.

In California, a long-haired teen practices his guitar and waits to hear from admissions at the college of his dreams. Music is his life, and he's excited to be a music major. He looks forward to living on campus, though he knows his parents will miss him. He's able to care for himself, even if laundry is something he hasn't quite mastered!

These young men all lead normal lives. And all three have hemophilia, a hereditary blood-clotting disorder: the same disorder your child has. All three are achievers. All three are actively engaged in life. And all three consider themselves normal kids.

WHAT ARE YOUR ASSOCIATIONS WITH HEMOPHILIA?

Associations are emotional or cognitive connections we all make to specific events, experiences, or objects. Hearing a certain song might make you smile, thinking of the summer when you fell in love and that song was played. Another song might make you feel strong, remembering when you once ran a race in record time while listening to it. When you learned that your child had hemophilia, what feelings, thoughts, images, or memories came to mind?

Many people who aren't familiar with hemophilia conjure terrifying images of sickly children, blood, pain, or isolation. But the reality of hemophilia is very different.

Consider another scene, in Michigan: summer camp. It's a warm day, and campers are down by the lake. The older ones know each other well after attending camp together for many years. They mentor and counsel the younger ones now. Deep bonds have formed among the campers because they understand each other, share similar needs, concerns, fears, and capabilities. What do they have in common? Everyone has hemophilia, and everyone is accepted. Even the camp counselors have hemophilia. The campers engage in many activities: archery, swimming, rock climbing, arts and crafts, boating, kayaking, woodworking, cooking. They feel sad when they must eventually pack up and go home. But they'll see their friends at future family gatherings through their local hemophilia organization.

Now, imagine a huge event in Texas: many parents arrive with their young children who have hemophilia. The kids are whisked off to daycare for the morning and then take a trip with experienced staff to the local zoo. For the adults, a guest speaker presents information about insurance. A social worker offers resources and advice. A nurse explains treatment options.

At midday, everyone breaks so the mothers can receive massages and the fathers can hang out together. The adults reconvene after lunch to talk and laugh together. New parents share their worries and receive counseling, consolation, and advice from experienced families. At the end of the day, everyone leaves with lots of knowledge and memories, and a sense that they now belong to a special community—

a family where everyone shares life with hemophilia, and everyone supports each other.

Does all this sound like hemophilia to you? Probably not. Why might we react initially with fear, and associate hemophilia with negative experiences? You'll learn why in the first chapter of this book.

It's time to create some new associations with hemophilia—empowering, optimistic ones. This book will help you do that. And it will give you the tools to reinforce positive associations throughout your child's development.

HEMOPHILIA NOW

Your child with hemophilia couldn't have been born at a better time. Products are safer, knowledge abounds, and treatment is advanced. We're raising a generation of children who have few complications and lead almost completely normal lives. Your child will probably lead this kind of life, too.

Today, the reality of hemophilia isn't what you think. Children are not in grave danger, will not be stigmatized, and won't even look different. The microscopic differences are in the blood. Yes, the reality is that your child will require shots. But the reality is also that shots—**infusions**—will become as much a part of your child's life as playtime, brushing teeth, and doing homework. Indeed, what seems difficult or scary at first eventually becomes routine. What seems impossible becomes achievable. Amazingly, what seems like a curse may one day seem like a blessing.

Hemophilia is an open door to a land where many families feel blessed by their children, privileged to have the excellent medical care they can receive in this country, and lucky to have such great support systems. Walk through this door, and see what they have seen:

- A young man with hemophilia who is a national karate champion
- A professional baseball player who has hemophilia
- Snowboarders, mountain bikers, rock climbers—all with hemophilia

- A university coach for a hockey team who has hemophilia
- Twins with hemophilia
- A girl with hemophilia
- A hematologist with hemophilia
- Men with hemophilia who marry and have children
- A family that willingly adopted a child with hemophilia
- Parents who have five children with hemophilia

There are superstars with hemophilia, and regular people with hemophilia living ordinary lives. Hemophilia isn't a reason to feel special or to feel cursed. It just is. This book will help you face the challenge and appreciate the wonder of hemophilia with confidence and knowledge.

The *wonder* of hemophilia? Yes. Hemophilia will help you discover something new about yourself: some potential, passion, or ability that you never knew you had. You may appreciate your child more. And you may value health, happiness, and home more.

But first, you must experience and learn new things. You're entering a new territory, exploring a new land that may seem scary at first. But you have this book as a map. And you have many physicians, advocates, and other families as guides to escort you safely on your journey. Welcome to the land of hemophilia, to our community, to our life. You're a part of us now, and we want you to feel secure, competent, and joyful. And you will!

∽ 1 ∾

"Your child has hemophilia."

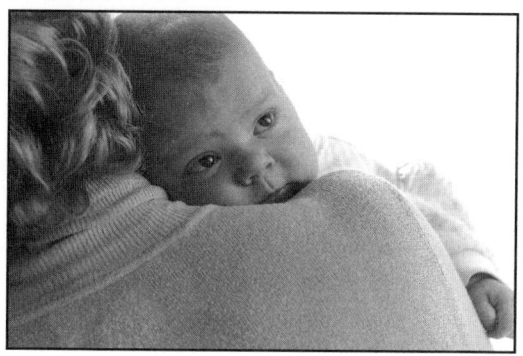

Although there was a feeling of loss [at the diagnosis], I was encouraged by two people's examples: my mother, who raised a child with a hearing impairment by learning a whole new language and teaching it to the family; and my grandmother, who had two boys with hemophilia back when there wasn't any treatment. I knew if they could do it, I could do it!
—Mary Fitzpatrick, New Hampshire

When you were pregnant and people asked if you wanted a boy or a girl, how many times did you say, "We just want a healthy baby"? Giving birth is one of life's special joys, and parents look forward to the big day with excitement, some anxiety, and even fear.

Why fear? We often fear the unknown or unexpected. And now that you've given birth, the thing you may have feared most has actually happened. Your doctor has informed you that your baby has a rare, chronic medical condition: "Your child has **hemophilia**." Hearing these words, you may feel stunned, shocked, scared. How could this obscure disorder have happened to your child? What is hemophilia?

Hemophilia is a rare, **genetic** blood-clotting disorder, affecting primarily males. Although it has existed throughout recorded history, hemophilia is often associated with late nineteenth- and early twentieth-century European kings and queens. It's mistakenly called the "royal disease." But in truth, anyone can be born with hemophilia, regardless of race, religion, or ethnicity. Yet most people never meet anyone with the disorder. Hemophilia often conjures up images of fragile, sick children who gush blood. These distorted, old-fashioned perceptions may be what you envision when you realize that this rare disorder has entered your life, your home, your baby.

As parents, you may struggle to accept hemophilia in your lives. You may wonder, "Where did this come from? How could this have happened to us?" And you may say, "We did nothing to deserve this!"

Fortunately, as you learn the facts about hemophilia and discover all the marvelous things that children with hemophilia can do, your worries will subside. As your confidence grows, you can focus again on the special joy of having a baby, raising a child. For now, you may experience a transition period when your fear of the unknown sometimes outweighs the truth that hemophilia is manageable and that your child can have a rich, full, normal life.

COMMON INITIAL FEELINGS

Childbirth is an emotional experience. Add the diagnosis of hemophilia, and it's normal for parents to experience a flood of turbulent emotions. Even when hemophilia is known to run in a family, the diagnosis may trigger intense feelings. Some parents deny the diagnosis, having convinced themselves that the inheritance would spare their child. Other parents grieve as they recall the suffering and pain of a hemophilic father or brother.

Many of our initial feelings have a common origin: the fear of losing control. Life hasn't gone as planned; the unexpected has suddenly happened. As adults, we strive for mastery in our lives. We choose where we live, we make friends, we vote, we manage our money, and we determine our careers. We can even choose when to have children.

But when we hear that our child has hemophilia, our sense of control seems shattered. We may feel like helpless victims of a crime. Something valuable has indeed been stolen: a sense of security about our baby's health. As parents, we want to protect and nurture our child, but hemophilia seems to threaten our ability to do that.

Two things gradually calm these rocketing emotions: information and experience. As you learn more about hemophilia, you'll regain control. You'll make better decisions when you understand treatment options. You won't feel afraid when your child bleeds, because you'll know what to do. And the more you experience hemophilia, the more confident you'll become. You'll learn what to expect, and you'll see how well you can handle it. Over time, hemophilia will be a normal, routine part of life.

To ease this transition, keep in mind that you are adjusting to a major life change. Any sudden life change—suffering a loss, changing careers, retiring, marrying, even winning the lottery—requires you to adjust your emotions and belief systems. And this takes time. So be good to yourself. Allow yourself space and time to experience the variety of emotions you feel. You'll work through them eventually, as you regain your balance and sense of control.

UNWANTED CHANGE: STAGES OF ACCEPTANCE

The most beautiful people we have known are those who have known defeat, known suffering, known struggle, known loss, and have found their way out of the depths. These persons have an appreciation, a sensitivity, and an understanding of life that fills them with compassion, gentleness, and a deep loving concern. Beautiful people do not just happen. —Dr. Elisabeth Kübler-Ross

For most parents, the hemophilia diagnosis signals an unwanted life change. It's irreversible, and it's frightening at first. As with any permanent life change, you'll need to work through your tumultuous feelings to reach emotional acceptance and peace of mind.

One way to do this is to identify your feelings. Sounds simple, doesn't it? But it isn't always easy to put a label on what you feel. Many parents go through stages of acceptance, a series of common emotions resulting from a loss or major life change. These are really stages of grieving, and they might happen when a loved one dies, a job is lost, a marriage ends, or a house burns down. With hemophilia, you are also grieving. Perhaps you've lost your dream of a "perfect" child or lost your sense of security about the future. You may feel a temporary loss of hope, faith, even joy.

The stages of acceptance outlined here are now a commonly recognized model in psychology. They originated with research on the grieving process by psychiatrist Elisabeth Kübler-Ross, MD, who interviewed the dying and their loved ones.[1] The model has expanded to include stages of acceptance of any major life change that involves loss. As you read through the stages, you may realize that you're feeling some of these emotions right now. Remember that you don't necessarily go through the stages in sequence, and you can experience some of them simultaneously. Some may be brief, and others may persist stubbornly. Where do you fit in?

Shock

Shock is emotional numbness. It's also called dissociation. Dissociation is a psychological defense. It protects you from sudden, overwhelming trauma that might leave you so emotionally paralyzed that you can't care for your baby or yourself. To allow you to keep functioning, at least superficially, your mind disconnects your emotions from the troubling event. Your emotions are there—but ignored, to be dealt with later. When you dissociate, you may have no strong initial reaction to the hemophilia diagnosis. You may shrug and think, "Oh, that's strange." Dissociation allows you to function: you can care for your child, cook dinner, or socialize superficially. But your ability to express emotions is temporarily limited.

1 *"Your child has hemophilia."*

Denial

Eventually, your body and emotions adjust, and shock wears off. You may experience denial: a powerful, normal defense mechanism that gives you a temporary feeling of control. When you're in denial, you think that this diagnosis is a mistake. You cuddle your beautiful baby and wonder how he could possibly have anything wrong with him. Denial creates an almost invisible, protective emotional barrier around you, pushing the problem outside. With the problem "out there," you don't have to deal with it. You have time to take a deep breath, cook dinner, feed and bathe the baby, watch television—and adjust to the diagnosis at a pace you can handle. You may think, "Those doctors don't know everything. He can't possibly have hemophilia. He looks just fine."

Denial may be even stronger if your child is diagnosed at a later age, perhaps after his first birthday. Denial can occur even when hemophilia is known to run in the family and when a mother knows she is a **carrier**.

Anger

Beyond denial, you may feel anger. You may think, "Why did this have to happen? It's not fair!" You may feel cheated out of a perfectly healthy baby. Your anger may be directed at God, Mother Nature, fate, your spouse or partner, even your doctor. If you already have one child with hemophilia, you might have believed that this was your turn to have a "normal" child. Or your anger may result from simply watching your baby endure bleeds and have necessary—but unpleasant—blood tests.

Anger may be born of frustration: you can't do anything to control events. Hemophilia is here to stay, and you can't change that. But anger is a normal reaction. It's a sign that you've started to give your emotions room to surface and expand, so you can begin to master them. Anger can be a positive sign that you're on the road to accepting hemophilia as a permanent part of your life, and that you're willing to start working with it. Share your emerging feelings with an experienced professional, like a social worker, if you feel that anger is becoming pervasive or harming your relationships with important people in your life.

Sadness

After your anger subsides, you may feel sadness. You may cry and feel hopeless. This is grief. You may grieve because your child has recently suffered from a blood test or a bleed. You may grieve because you think he will lose the carefree childhood he deserves. You may grieve for the joy you might have shared. "This is terrible," you may think. "My poor baby! How will we handle this?" Yet your sadness is a sign that you are accepting the diagnosis.[2]

Guilt

When you hear the diagnosis of hemophilia, it's normal to want to blame something or someone. Psychologically, you want to assign responsibility for this unexpected event. Why? Because this might make you feel a temporary sense of control, and because in truth, it's not your fault. Unfortunately, if you choose to blame yourself, you may feel tremendous guilt.

Mothers may feel guilt because most often, it's the mother who transmits hemophilia to her child. If a mother is a carrier of the hemophilia **gene**, she may feel responsible for passing along this "bad" gene to her child.[3] A mother may wonder, "Did I give this to him?" Even mothers who aren't carriers may feel twinges of guilt, and some take full responsibility for the disorder, as if they caused it willfully.

Do fathers ever feel guilty? Of course. Society expects boys to be physically active and competitive. A father may feel disappointed when his son has a blood-clotting disorder that he mistakenly thinks will limit physical ability, making his child physically vulnerable. And because the father's **chromosomes** determine the sex of the child (see Chapter 2), fathers may be prey to guilt.

Feelings of guilt are normal, even though rationally we know that the occurrence of hemophilia can't be controlled. Can you control your child's eye color? Hair color? Height? Of course not! True, your child may have hemophilia because of your gene, but you did not choose to be a carrier or transmit this disorder. Nothing you did during your pregnancy—too much exercise, alcohol, stress, smoking—caused it. Whether willed by God, decided by fate, or the result of a random genetic **mutation**, your child has hemophilia for reasons beyond your control.

Identifying your stage of acceptance, and knowing why you're there, can help you master your emotions and regain emotional stability as you move toward accepting the diagnosis. The key is to recognize that you are in a certain stage, but you're progressing. Acknowledge the stage, feel the emotions associated with it, move to the next stage when you're ready, and keep moving toward acceptance. If you are stuck in a stage too long, your family will suffer. Your baby with hemophilia needs you. With acceptance will come balance, perspective, and the return of joy.

FATHERS AND MOTHERS: DIFFERING REACTIONS

Hemophilia can be a source of great stress, and people cope with stress in various ways. Some experts believe that men and women process stress differently. So when a mother and father turn to each other for support after hearing the diagnosis, one parent may be surprised when the other reacts in a less-than-supportive manner. One seems too emotional, the other too distant. It's not unusual for a father and mother to react differently to their child's diagnosis—in fact, it's normal.

One reason that parents' reactions may differ is that they simply are different people. Are you the openly emotional type, or are you the reserved, task-oriented type? Are you the nurturing type or the pull-yourself-up-by-the-bootstraps type?

Another reason for gender differences in emotional response is centuries of biological conditioning. As males and females, our evolutionary biological hardwiring differs. From hormones to muscle mass, from memory to mental processing, our differences work to preserve the human species. Add to that centuries of cultural conditioning, and males and females have learned to enact very different roles.

Mothers traditionally tend to be more relational. They take on emotional processing for the family. A mother may express her emotions: crying, talking openly about hemophilia, or worrying greatly. The empathetic attention she receives from friends and family comforts her temporarily and distracts her from stress. Her intense feelings may also lead her to enmesh herself emotionally in a family problem; healthy emotional boundaries that separate her from other family members may blur.

Fathers are generally oriented toward achievements and goals. They want to be rational problem solvers or heroes. To a father, hemophilia is a problem affecting his family, and maybe he can solve it. To do this, he may withdraw emotionally for a while, not showing his feelings. He may focus more on medical facts than on emotions, appearing strong and stoic. Or he may distance himself from his feelings by attending more to work, hobbies, and sports than to the family.

A father's stoicism doesn't mean that he doesn't feel. One mother recalls, "Sure, I cried and he was the strong one—so I thought. Years later, he told me that he secretly struggled with depression but felt that he needed to be strong for me." Both parents experience the full range of emotions, yet may express them in different ways.

If fathers and mothers don't understand how their partner copes

1 *"Your child has hemophilia."*

with stress, they may experience tension, resentment, conflict, or distancing. For example, a mother may not understand that the hemophilia diagnosis can rob a man of his feelings of confidence and competence. The mother may feel hurt or resentful if he withdraws from her. To her, he isn't withdrawing just to seek a solution—he seems to be removing emotional support from her at a time when she needs it most.

A father may not understand that the diagnosis can cause a woman to seek comfort through relationships. She may work out her feelings by talking. She may spend more time away from him, with other family members or friends. The father may feel neglected, not realizing that instead of a solution to the problem, she may need reassurance, sympathy, and validation of her feelings. She needs to be heard.

How can a relationship weather the diagnosis of hemophilia? When parents understand the way each partner copes with stress, they become more respectful of each other's needs and can respond appropriately and lovingly to meet those needs. Here's how you can help your spouse or partner at this difficult time:

- Expect that fathers and mothers may react differently—not only because of gender differences, but because they are different people.
- Try not to take reactions personally. A father's emotional withdrawal doesn't mean he doesn't care. A mother's prolonged crying doesn't mean she is having a breakdown.
- Remember that people go through stages of acceptance at varying rates. The father might be in denial when the mother has moved on to anger. Remind yourself that stages usually pass, and that your partner will soon move on at his or her own pace, while receiving support and compassion.

Stages of acceptance can take anywhere from a few weeks to months, or even years. Advancing through the stages may take longer if parents are stuck in their own stages and don't respect or support each other's particular way of coping. If negative emotions—anger, depression, dissociation—seem to persist for months, parents should consider some form of counseling. A child with hemophilia needs emotionally stable, reliable parents who are able to work through periods of stress. A counselor can help ease friction between parents and speed the process of regaining control over everyday life, so the child gets the best care.

CHANGE YOUR FOCUS

Positive expectations spring from hope and from the belief that we can control much of what happens in our lives. Dashed expectations are a major reason that parents react to the diagnosis with denial, anger, or sadness. After months of preparation for the birth of a "healthy" child, you suddenly find yourself unprepared, uneducated about hemophilia, and dependent on doctors. You may question your beliefs about life and faith. One way to regain your sense of control is to change your focus. Try to focus on things you can control, not on things you can't. You can change your focus in two ways:

1. Ask *how* questions, not *why* questions. Some parents focus on why their child has hemophilia. An answer may bring comfort to some: "Our child is special, and we are special to raise him," or "This will make us more compassionate people." But if you find yourself repeatedly asking "Why?" and not feeling comfort or finding answers, you need to ask instead, "How can I . . . ?"

Negative *why* questions	Positive *how* questions
"Why does my child have hemophilia?"	"How can I learn more about hemophilia?"
"Why do I feel so depressed?"	"How can I find some other people for support?"
"Why is nothing going right?"	"How can I feel better right now?"

1 "Your child has hemophilia."

Asking *why* questions can reinforce negative feelings. Asking *how* questions usually leads to action and answers.

2. Focus on your ability to take action—something you can control. Ask yourself, "What can I do right now to make things better?" You can pick up the phone and call someone. You can order information on hemophilia. You can admit that you're scared or anxious. You can also be careful how you phrase questions you ask yourself and others.

You can train your mind to focus on positive things that will empower you and restore your sense of control. Here's how:

- Try not to make comparisons that focus on everyone else's healthy child. Avoid asking, "Why isn't my sister's child afflicted with a medical condition? Why only mine?"
- Don't focus on the one thing that's "wrong" with your child. If you single out hemophilia, asking why he has this disorder, you are choosing not to acknowledge the millions of things right with your child.

THE HEMOPHILIA TREATMENT CENTER

Once you have accepted that your child has hemophilia, you may crave information to reinforce your new sense of control. To stay informed,

- Read books, brochures, and newsletters about hemophilia.
- Speak with professionals and experienced parents.

And of course, having a few experiences of your own with hemophilia will make you feel more competent.

Start gathering information and advice from your comprehensive **hemophilia treatment center (HTC)**. HTCs are medical centers of excellence that specialize in diagnosing and treating bleeding disorders. The physician who diagnosed your child may be able to refer you to the nearest center.[4] There are at least 140 centers in the United States, and most are affiliated with a major teaching hospital.

Most are located in urban centers, so families living in rural areas may not have easy access to a center. If you live far from an HTC, know that although local hospital staff might be able to treat your child's bleeds, they usually lack knowledge and experience with hemophilia and can't provide the in-depth care available at an HTC.

The HTC has a **multidisciplinary team** of medical specialists to treat the family and patient as a whole. The focus isn't solely on treating individual bleeding episodes, but on offering acute and long-term care, family and genetic counseling, surgery, education, physical therapy, and medical supplies specific to hemophilia patients.

Most HTCs have social workers on staff to help you work through your feelings about the diagnosis. They offer marriage counseling and help you with insurance problems. You will be assigned a **hematologist**[5] (a doctor who specializes in blood disorders) and a **nurse specialist** to educate you and give your child regular checkups. At your first visit, HTC staff will want to schedule blood tests to rule out other types of blood deficiencies and confirm the original diagnosis. You'll receive a lot of information, but don't expect to digest it all at once. At first, the doctors may sound like they're speaking a foreign language, and it takes time to feel comfortable with the new terminology.

You may be surprised at how little you remember of what you were told when your child was first diagnosed, and how much you can remember as the months progress. Your ability to retain information may reflect your acceptance of the diagnosis and your readiness to learn. Earlier, you may have been too overwhelmed, shocked, or sad to absorb much. Now you'll see that the more you learn, the better equipped you are to handle your emotions.

SUPPORT FROM OTHER PARENTS

You'll get some of the best everyday information from other parents. Your HTC or local hemophilia organization may already have a support

1   "Your child has hemophilia."

group that meets regularly, or you may want to start your own. Leave your contact information with your HTC or local organization so interested parents can get in touch. Internet chat groups and mailing lists allow parents to ask questions and share experiences.

From other parents, you'll receive advice on what to expect at different ages, as well as practical tips to prevent injuries. You'll meet parents who listen while you vent your worries and who share your deepest concerns. At support groups, you'll meet children with hemophilia and see for yourself that they don't have to be padded from head to toe to prevent bleeds. You'll be amazed at all the things these children can do and how normal life can become. Most of all, you'll observe other families living their lives—normally. When you become a welcomed member of a community, you'll feel less isolated, more accepted, and perfectly ordinary![6]

Of all the things you'll learn from other parents, the most important is that you are not alone. Some families are going through what you're experiencing now, and others have already been there. You'll probably leave a meeting or online chat feeling that life is more manageable. You'll begin to regain that sense of control.

GET SMART!

Parents today have access to information as never before. E-mail, Internet, and the Web offer nearly every American family the opportunity to log on and search for hemophilia information. Within seconds, families have access to websites, glossaries, treatment information, names, and phone numbers.

You'll find a tremendous amount of literature about hemophilia: books, booklets, DVDs, CDs for children, siblings, and parents. Look at the resource list in Appendix A. You only have to call, fax, write, or email for information on a variety of subjects. Discuss this information with your nurse or hematologist at your HTC, and get your questions answered.

The only problem you may have is that you feel overwhelmed by so much worthwhile information! Here's a short list of contacts to begin:

- **National Hemophilia Foundation (NHF)**
  800-42-HANDI
  www.hemophilia.org
- **Hemophilia Federation of America (HFA)**
  800-230-9797
  www.hemophiliafed.org
- **Your local hemophilia organization**
- **LA Kelley Communications, Inc.**
  978-352-7657
  www.kelleycom.com
- **Free resources** (Appendix A)
- **The website of your child's factor manufacturer** (see Appendix B)

Read one article, chapter, or webpage about hemophilia a day. Don't get overwhelmed by trying to absorb too much. Pace yourself.

Exploring all these educational materials will make you feel better. You'll have more control, and you'll be prepared and informed. Knowledge helps you make better decisions and become an involved, active parent. From a worried, helpless bystander, you'll develop into a powerful **advocate** for your child: you'll be able to tell doctors, nurses, teachers, and in-laws what you need when you need it. As a result, your child will receive the best available care and the best available products, provided by the best available mom or dad—that's you!

1 "Your child has hemophilia."

"Your child has hemophilia."
Chapter 1 Summary

- When you receive your child's diagnosis, it's normal for you to experience a range of intense feelings, from shock to denial, from anger to sadness.
- Expect that you and your partner or spouse may react differently to the diagnosis.
- Information and experience will help you feel you have more control.
- Change your focus on things you can't control to things you can control.
- At least 140 HTCs specialize in treating children and adults with hemophilia and their families. Contact the one near you.
- Contact other parents of children with hemophilia through your HTC or local hemophilia organization.
- Read everything you can about hemophilia, at a pace that makes you comfortable. You'll develop options and confidence, and you'll make better decisions.
- Use the Internet to search for hemophilia information from respected websites. Start with these:
  www.hemophilia.org
  www.hemophiliafed.org
  www.kelleycom.com

2

What Is Hemophilia?

No, my child will not bleed to death with a cut. No, he will not grow out of hemophilia. Yes, he gets poked several times a week, and then he can be normal just like your child. Yes, that's my child climbing a tree, riding a scooter, playing a sport. We have hemophilia. It doesn't have us!
—Vanessa Stowers Flora, Indiana

Before your child was born, hemophilia may have been vaguely familiar to you. Something to do with bleeding? Some connection to European royalty? You may not know much about hemophilia unless it runs in your family. Yet in one-third of diagnosed hemophilia cases, there is no family history. Hemophilia's sudden appearance may be the biggest surprise of your life.

Hemophilia is a genetic disorder that prevents blood from forming an effective clot. Without effective blood clotting, bleeding may be prolonged or not stop. This can cause joint damage or other complications, and may be life-threatening. Although hemophilia follows no racial or geographic pattern, it occurs almost exclusively in males. Hemophilia is rare: it's estimated that only about 20,000 people in the United States have hemophilia. **Hemophilia A** occurs in approximately 1 in 5,000 male births. **Hemophilia B** occurs in about 1 in 20,000 male births.[1] To put this in perspective, Down **syndrome** occurs in 1 of every 700 births, and spina bifida occurs in 1 to 2 of every 1,000 births. Although rare, hemophilia can happen not only to kings and princes, but to anyone, including you.

MYTHS

Perhaps because hemophilia is so rare, it has generated many myths. Myths are stories, sometimes created by people in an attempt to make something understandable when scientific information is unavailable. Remember the Greek tale of Pandora's Box? Pandora was the first woman on earth. She was given a wedding gift from the gods, a beautiful container. But she was warned never to open it. Driven by curiosity, she disobeyed the gods and opened it. Inside were evils—hate, disease, pain—that flew out of the container and escaped into the world. This story was invented by the ancient Greeks to explain sickness and suffering, because they didn't know about bacteria and viruses. Some myths develop from a nugget of fact or experience, but then take on a life of their own within certain cultural settings.

Becoming familiar with the most widely held myths about hemophilia and their sources will help you explain the facts of the disorder to others. Here are some common myths about hemophilia.

Myth: Hemophilia is a royal disease.
Truth: Anyone can get hemophilia—rich or poor, famous or unknown. Hemophilia was dubbed the royal disease because in the 1800s, hemophilia affected the family of Queen Victoria of England, who was a carrier of the hemophilia gene. Hemophilia was transmitted to three other royal families when Victoria's daughters and granddaughters, also carriers, married into the Russian, German, and Spanish royal families. Though it's no longer known to be present in any European royal family, hemophilia is still often associated with royalty.

Myth: A small cut will cause blood to rush out, and the child will bleed to death.
Truth: People with hemophilia do not bleed faster than anyone else. But they will bleed longer because their blood doesn't clot properly. Still, not every cut will continue to bleed just because a person has hemophilia. Some cuts, especially small ones, stop bleeding on their own.

2 What Is Hemophilia?

Myth: Children with hemophilia cannot play sports.
Truth: Children with hemophilia enjoy a wide variety of sports, including swimming, baseball, tennis, running, and martial arts. You'll realize this someday when you're chauffeuring your sports fan to various afterschool activities! High-impact contact sports such as football, hockey, and boxing are not advised. Physical activity is always encouraged for children with hemophilia.

Myth: Children with hemophilia must wear helmets and protective gear.
Truth: Although some parents place protective helmets or knee pads on their toddlers, it's uncommon for a child with hemophilia to wear protective gear for normal activities. Medical treatments today are excellent and easy, offering a normal lifestyle. Of course, all children must wear protective gear when participating in risky activities: helmets should always be worn when riding bikes or motorcycles, or when skiing or snowboarding. Oh yes, your child will be able to do these things one day!

Myth: Children with hemophilia must attend a special needs school.
Truth: Except for having a defective blood protein for blood clotting, our children have normal health and intelligence. They can be enrolled in any school. Overall, your child is normal and will be treated as such by the school system and the public.

Myth: Children with hemophilia will grow out of it.
Truth: Hemophilia is a lifelong condition. Your child does not have a disease that will get better or go into remission. Your child will not grow out of hemophilia: the mechanism for producing **clotting factor** is defective. Hemophilia is part of his genetic makeup, just like traits for hair or eye color, which can't be outgrown.[2]

Myth: Hemophilia causes **AIDS**.
Truth: Hemophilia does not cause **acquired immune deficiency syndrome** (AIDS). People with hemophilia are no more susceptible than anyone else to the **human immunodeficiency virus** (HIV) infection

that causes AIDS. HIV is transmitted through body fluids, including blood. Almost 90% of people with **severe hemophilia** contracted HIV between 1978 and 1985 after receiving **factor concentrate** derived from HIV-tainted blood donations. Since March 1985, all blood donors are screened for HIV risk factors and donations are tested for the presence of HIV. But no blood test is perfect. As an added **safety** measure, blood-derived factor concentrates are also treated to inactivate or destroy HIV and most other viruses (see Appendix D). Today, hemophilia treatments are available that contain no blood-derived proteins.

Myth: Hemophilia is caused by something you did during pregnancy.
Truth: Nothing you did while pregnant gave your baby hemophilia. Women who have perfect pregnancies and follow every safety precaution can give birth to children with hemophilia. There's nothing you could have done to prevent hemophilia; nor could you have changed your child's hair or eye color. Hemophilia is simply part of his genetic makeup.

Have you have heard some of these hemophilia myths? You'll feel better knowing that, like the story of Pandora's Box, people believed these myths when they lacked facts. This chapter will give you the facts!

HOW BLOOD CLOTS

To understand hemophilia, you must understand a little about blood. Blood is a life-giving liquid that travels throughout your body in tubes called blood vessels. There are three kinds of blood vessels: **arteries**, **veins**, and **capillaries**. When you take a breath, your heart pumps freshly oxygenated blood to your body through the arteries. The arteries deliver blood to the capillaries, the tiniest blood vessels, bringing food and oxygen to cells throughout your body. Cells then exchange the food and oxygen for cellular waste products such as carbon dioxide. This oxygen-poor blood, now carrying carbon dioxide,

2 What Is Hemophilia?

returns to your heart through your veins. Your heart then pumps this "used" blood to the lungs, where your blood exchanges its load of carbon dioxide for oxygen. Each time you breathe, you exhale carbon dioxide and breathe in oxygen, helping the blood do its job.

Blood has four main components:

- **Plasma**, a yellowish fluid that comprises about 55% of the blood volume
- Red blood cells, which carry oxygen and carbon dioxide
- White blood cells, which defend the body from bacteria, viruses, and other foreign invaders
- **Platelets**, cells that help form blood clots in damaged blood vessels

Blood cells have a limited lifespan and are continually being replaced. If you lose some blood through a torn blood vessel, your body replaces it by producing more.

What exactly happens when you lose blood?

When a blood vessel is cut or torn, blood leaks out. The damaged blood vessel sends out chemical signals that an injury has occurred. These chemical signals initiate a process called **hemostasis** to limit the blood loss, and this culminates with the marvelous, complex **clotting cascade**, which forms a blood clot. Hemostasis happens in three stages:

1. Vasoconstriction. Muscles in the damaged blood vessel wall tighten, narrowing its diameter and reducing blood flow inside the injured vessel. Even in people with hemophilia, vasoconstriction in blood vessels may sometimes be enough to stop blood flow from small cuts.

2. Platelet plug. Platelets are activated at the site of the injury, causing them to become sticky and adhere to the wound and to each other. The sticky platelets plug the hole in the blood vessel.

3. Fibrin clot. The platelet plug is weak. To prevent it from breaking down and falling out, restarting the bleeding, the plug must be strengthened and held in place. This is done with **fibrin**, a tough fibrous substance produced by a complex reaction of plasma proteins called clotting factors. Clotting factors travel in the bloodstream. There are at least thirteen clotting factors, each identified by a roman numeral (factor I, factor II, factor III, and so on). When chemically activated, by signals from a damaged blood vessel and later by the platelets, the factors all work together in the clotting cascade in sequence. Each factor is responsible for a specific step in the formation of fibrin fibers, eventually making a network of tough threads that weave themselves through the platelet plug, strengthening and holding it in place, making a fibrin clot (see Fig. 2.1).

Once the fibrin clot is formed, the healing process begins. New cells can then form to repair the torn blood vessel. When healing is completed, the fibrin clot is reabsorbed into the blood, or it falls off externally as a scab.[3]

WHY DOES YOUR CHILD CONTINUE TO BLEED?

Having hemophilia means that the body can't produce a strong fibrin clot. Without fibrin to strengthen and hold the weak platelet plug in place, the plug is easily broken and falls out, and blood continues to leak.

The body can't produce a strong fibrin clot when one of the clotting factors is missing or inactive—"inactive" means the factor is actually present but doesn't function correctly. Remember, when a blood vessel is torn and blood leaks out, chemicals released into the bloodstream trigger a sequence of events: (1) vasoconstriction, (2) a platelet plug, and through the clotting cascade, (3) a fibrin clot. If just one of the clotting factors is missing or inactive, the reaction may stop and fibrin will not be produced.

Think of the clotting cascade as a relay race, with each factor handing instructions to the next factor. If one of the runners isn't there

2 What Is Hemophilia?

Fig. 2.1 **How Blood Clots**

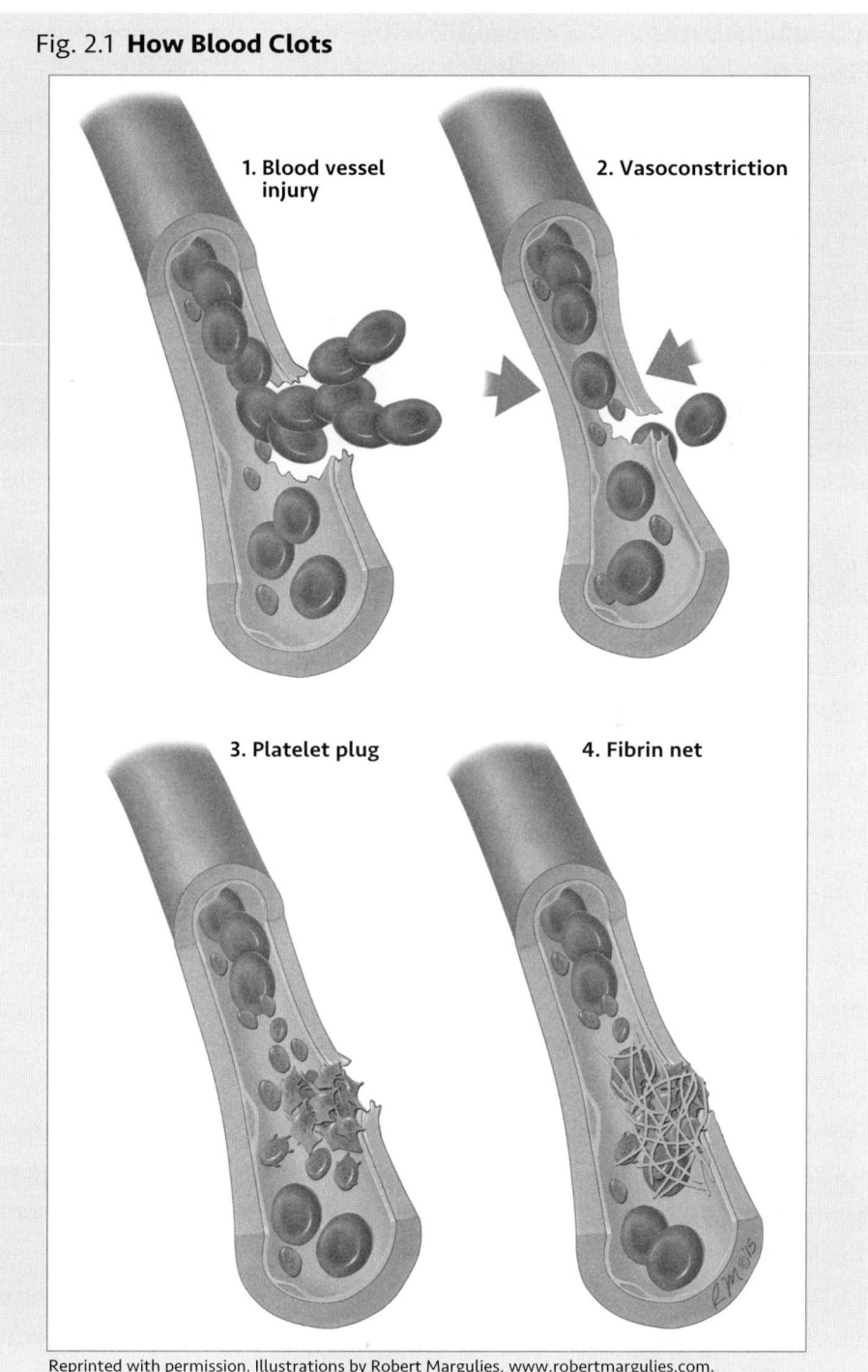

Reprinted with permission. Illustrations by Robert Margulies, www.robertmargulies.com.

to grab instructions from the previous runner, the instructions are dropped, and the race to make a fibrin clot is never completed.

Which type of hemophilia does your child have? That is, which clotting factor is your child missing?

Factor VIII. If your child lacks factor VIII, he has factor VIII deficiency, or hemophilia A (also called classical hemophilia). This is the most common factor deficiency, affecting about 80% of people with hemophilia.

Factor IX. If your child lacks factor IX, he has factor IX deficiency, or hemophilia B. This is the second most common factor deficiency, affecting about 20% of people with hemophilia. Hemophilia B is also called **Christmas disease**, named after Stephen Christmas, a 10-year-old boy from England who in 1952 was the first person to be diagnosed with hemophilia B.

People can have hemophilia if they lack other clotting factors besides factor VIII and factor IX, but this is extremely rare. While your child is being tested for his hemophilia type, he will probably also be tested for another bleeding disorder: **von Willebrand disease** (VWD). VWD is the most common inherited bleeding disorder, possibly existing in 1% to 3% of the human population.[4]

It's important to know which type of factor deficiency your child has, because this will determine his treatment.

HOW SEVERE IS YOUR CHILD'S HEMOPHILIA?

Just as you need to know your child's hemophilia type, you must also know his **severity level**. Severity level is a measure, usually described as a range, of the amount of factor active in the bloodstream (the factor level). So your child will be diagnosed first by type of hemophilia (factor VIII, IX, or other) and then by severity level. He may have **severe, moderate,** or **mild hemophilia.** Your hematologist might tell you your child is "severe factor VIII deficient" or has "mild hemophilia B." There are technical and practical differences among the factor levels that will influence what treatment he receives.[5]

Severe hemophilia: less than 1% of factor active
Moderate hemophilia: 1% to 5% of factor active
Mild hemophilia: 6% to 50% of factor active

The good news is that if your child has mild or moderate hemophilia, he might have some factor working in his blood, possibly enough to make a clot. Severity levels are **hereditary**: if his relative has severe hemophilia, your child's hemophilia will be severe, too. Severity levels do not change. If your child tests as severe, moderate, or mild, he will always test that way.

What are normal factor levels? Among the general population, normal factor levels are between 50% and 150%, with most people being close to 100%. Factor VIII levels can vary and are affected by some hormones. For example, factor VIII levels may rise in pregnant women, when a person is scared or stressed, or after vigorous exercise (factor IX levels do not change with pregnancy, hormones, or after stress or exercise).

People whose factor levels are at the higher end of the mild hemophilia range (between 25% and 50% of factor active) may not show unusual bleeding tendencies unless subjected to trauma, even though their levels are below normal. Some people with mild hemophilia may not be diagnosed until they have excessive bleeding resulting from trauma. But remember: some people with factor in these ranges *do* experience bleeds. And women who are carriers of the hemophilia gene (see page 33) often have factor levels in the mild hemophilia range, and may have prolonged bleeding and bleeding from trauma. Carriers should have their factor level tested and, if it's low, should have a treatment plan ready in case they suffer trauma and begin bleeding excessively.

SPEAKING PRACTICALLY: SEVERITY LEVELS AND BLEEDING

What does all this mean in practical terms for your child? Although every child with hemophilia is different, there are general trends in how people with different severity levels will bleed:

- Children with severe hemophilia can bleed spontaneously (with no apparent injury), usually into joints, in addition to having bleeds from injuries.
- Children with mild or moderate hemophilia rarely have spontaneous bleeds, but instead usually bleed from an injury or from surgical or dental procedures.

Usually, but not always, children with severe hemophilia bleed more often than children with mild or moderate hemophilia. Another practical aspect of severity level is how often your child will bleed. If not on prophylaxis (regular infusions of factor concentrate to prevent bleeds) and not using longer-acting factor concentrates, children with severe hemophilia may bleed from 20 to over 100 times per year. Moderately affected children may bleed only once a month or once a year. Mildly affected children may bleed only rarely, usually as a result of trauma or surgery.

Today, many children with severe hemophilia infuse clotting factor to *prevent* bleeds. This is called **prophylaxis**. Prophylaxis is the scheduled infusion of factor concentrate, designed to keep some factor in the blood at all times. The goal is to prevent spontaneous (not due to trauma) joint bleeds and the resulting joint damage.[6] Prophylaxis can be so effective that some children with hemophilia on "prophy" have never had a joint bleed!

Although people with severe hemophilia usually bleed more often than those with mild or moderate hemophilia, this may vary significantly from person to person. Some children with severe hemophilia rarely bleed, while some with moderate hemophilia bleed regularly. Over time, you'll learn your child's bleeding tendencies. And, in cooperation with his hematologist, you'll learn how to tailor your child's therapy to his specific bleeding tendencies. The goal is to treat bleeds effectively, and also to prevent **spontaneous bleeds**. Doctors will rely on your expertise because you know your child best.

HOW BLEEDING IS TREATED

People with mild or moderate hemophilia A have some functional factor VIII circulating in their blood. Factor VIII and IX are produced primarily in the liver, although the cells lining the blood vessels also hold reserves of factor VIII for release into the bloodstream when needed. A drug called **desmopressin acetate** can trigger the release of some of these factor reserves, temporarily boosting circulating factor levels up to twice their usual levels. Depending on the initial factor level, this boost in factor levels may be enough to control a minor bleed and avoid an infusion.

In children with severe hemophilia—or to control major bleeds in children with mild or moderate hemophilia—the missing or inactive factor VIII or IX must be replaced. The most common and effective method is called *factor replacement therapy*, in which commercially prepared factor concentrate is infused into a vein. Once factor is infused, the normal chain of events that leads to clotting and formation of a strong fibrin clot can occur.

Children with factor VIII deficiency receive factor VIII replacement therapy. Children with factor IX deficiency receive factor IX replacement therapy.

What's an infusion?

An infusion is the injection of a drug into a vein. This is also called an **intravenous** infusion or IV infusion. Factor replacement therapy uses commercially prepared clotting factor, which comes in a vial as a freeze-dried powder ready for **reconstitution** (mixing) with the diluent—**sterile** water or sterile saline (salt water). After the factor is mixed with the diluent, it's drawn into a **syringe**. Then the factor is infused through a small **butterfly needle** inserted into your child's vein (called **venipuncture**) or through a **port** (a surgically implanted device connected to a vein). The factor is infused, or pushed in, through the syringe. After the infusion, direct pressure is held on the infusion site for 5 to 10 minutes to allow for clotting. An adhesive bandage may be applied at the infusion site to absorb any oozing blood. Treating hemophilia with factor concentrate is convenient and fast!

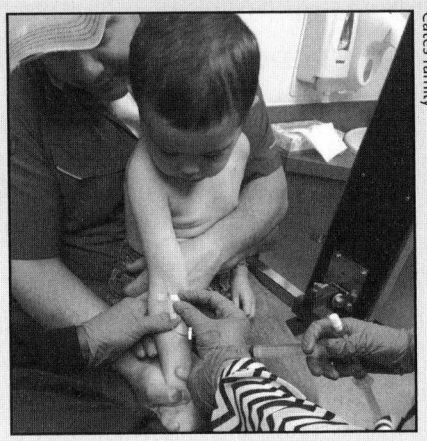

After standard factor is infused, it starts working immediately but stays in the bloodstream for only a short time—hours to days, depending on the type of factor. Even when factor is produced normally, in the liver or linings of blood vessels, and is released into the bloodstream, it's quickly used up, or degraded. Factor is like food: an "infusion" of one meal doesn't satisfy your appetite forever or give you boundless energy. Food is used up hours later, and you must eat more.

The body uses up factor like food and must replenish it. This explains why a whole blood transfusion from a person with normal factor production into a person with hemophilia won't cure hemophilia. The factor present in the normal blood would eventually be degraded in the body of the recipient with hemophilia, and would

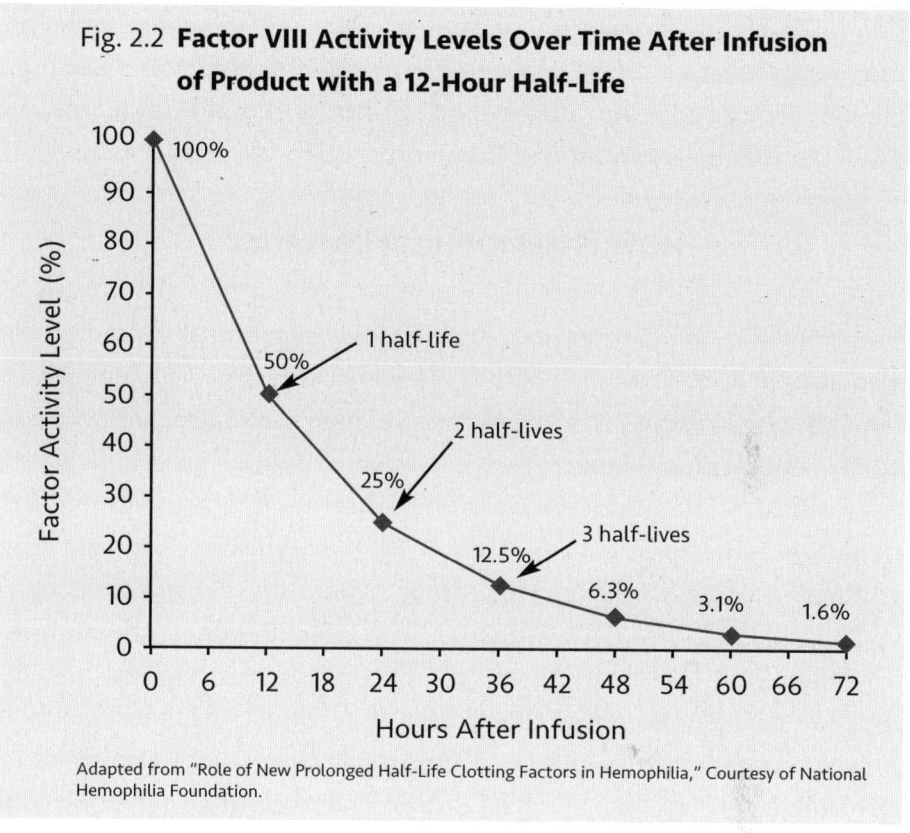

Fig. 2.2 **Factor VIII Activity Levels Over Time After Infusion of Product with a 12-Hour Half-Life**

Adapted from "Role of New Prolonged Half-Life Clotting Factors in Hemophilia," Courtesy of National Hemophilia Foundation.

need to be replenished. People without hemophilia can replace their factor naturally, but people with hemophilia can't. So an infusion doesn't cure them.

How long does factor last in the bloodstream? The length of time factor lasts is measured by its **half-life**, or the time it takes for one-half of the clotting activity to disappear. The average half-life of standard factor VIII is about 12 hours, usually less in children. (Individual half-lives vary from person to person and may range from as few as 4 hours to as many as 20 hours.) This means that close to 100% of the infused factor VIII is active, or able to help form a clot, when first infused. But over the next 12 hours, its activity steadily decreases to only 50% (see Figure 2.2).

Factor VIII continues to lose about 50% of its activity every 12 hours. So after 24 hours, only about 25% is active; at 36 hours, only about 12% activity remains, and so on. Factor IX has a longer half-life, about 24 hours. To ensure a secure clot after a major injury, several infusions may be given over several days to keep your child's factor levels high. Newer factor concentrates—called **prolonged half-life** factor—are available that have longer half-lives and require fewer infusions.

HOW IS HEMOPHILIA INHERITED?

Hemophilia is an inherited trait just like hair, eye, and skin color. It can also appear spontaneously, with no family history. How is it inherited in families with a history? Why does it occur mainly in males, and why only some males within a family?

First, let's talk about genetics. Inherited traits are determined by genes. A gene is a sequence of **DNA** (deoxyribonucleic acid) that contains a code for making a protein. Within the nucleus of each of your 3 trillion body cells are 20,000 to 25,000 genes, all grouped together on long strands called chromosomes. Genes are the biochemical blueprints of the body. They direct the production of proteins, which in turn direct all the major body processes. Proteins determine your eye, hair, and skin color. They also determine how your organs develop and function, how your bones grow, what you look like, and how well your blood clots. When a gene that's supposed to contain instructions for producing a key biological protein is damaged or missing, the result may be a genetic disorder like hemophilia.

There are 46 chromosomes in each of your body's cells, arranged in 23 pairs. (The exceptions are red blood cells, which have no chromosomes, and sex cells—egg and sperm—which each contain only 23 chromosomes.) Two of these 46 chromosomes are called the sex chromosomes, identified as X or Y. They are called sex chromosomes because together, these two chromosomes determine whether the baby will be male or female. Girls have two **X chromosomes**, and boys have one X and one **Y chromosome**.

Because the genes for producing factor VIII and factor IX are both found on the X chromosome, hemophilia is called an X-linked

2 What Is Hemophilia?

recessive disorder. These disorders affect primarily males because males have only one X chromosome. Mutations to the gene for either factor VIII or factor IX will result in hemophilia A or hemophilia B, respectively. For simplicity, we'll refer to mutations in either of these two genes as the "hemophilia gene."

If you're a carrier of the hemophilia gene, here's how the gene found its way into your child:

- A child is conceived when the sperm fertilizes the egg.
- The sperm contains 23 chromosomes—copies of one-half of the father's genetic makeup.
- The egg contains 23 chromosomes—copies of one-half of the mother's genetic makeup.
- When the sperm fertilizes the egg, the new embryo contains 46 chromosomes—half from the father, half from the mother.
- The egg always contributes an X chromosome.
- The sperm contributes either an X or a Y chromosome, and this determines the child's sex.
- A female is created when both the sperm and egg contribute X chromosomes. All females are XX.
- A male is created when the sperm contributes a Y chromosome and the egg contributes an X chromosome. All males are XY.
- The hemophilia gene is on an X chromosome.

If one of the inherited X chromosomes carries the hemophilia gene, then

- the girl will be a carrier of the hemophilia gene (one X not affected, one X affected), or
- the boy will have hemophilia (Y not affected, X affected).

A mother who is a carrier of hemophilia may not have bleeding problems. Why? Only one of a carrier mother's two X chromosomes contains the hemophilia gene. Her other chromosome contains a functional gene for clotting factor. As long as one chromosome provides correct instructions for making factor, enough factor is usually produced to compensate for the lack of factor caused by the hemophilia gene.[7]

When a male baby receives an affected X chromosome from his mother, he will have hemophilia. Why? As a male, he has an X and a Y chromosome. Because he has only one X from his mother, and that X carries the hemophilia gene, he has no unaffected backup X containing the correct instructions for producing functional clotting factor.

Just because you are a carrier, this doesn't mean you'll automatically give birth to a child with hemophilia! If you're a carrier, each of your children has a 50% chance of receiving an X chromosome containing the hemophilia gene. If you have a son, this means he has a 50% chance of having hemophilia. If you have a daughter, she has a 50% chance of being a carrier. It's like the flip of a coin: heads, it's a boy; tails, it's a girl. If it's a boy, flip again: heads, he has hemophilia; tails, he doesn't (see Fig. 2.3).

What happens when your son with hemophilia has children? He will contribute either an X or a Y chromosome to create an embryo. Every X chromosome from the father with hemophilia has the hemophilia gene, so *all* his daughters will be carriers of hemophilia. Every Y is normal, so *all* his sons will be unaffected. If he has only sons, hemophilia will disappear from his direct ancestry.

Do girls ever get hemophilia? You bet. A father with hemophilia and a carrier mother can produce a girl with hemophilia. In this case, there is a 50% chance that each daughter and son of this couple will have hemophilia:

- The father with hemophilia gives an X chromosome that carries the hemophilia gene.
- The carrier mother gives an X chromosome that carries the hemophilia gene.

In rare cases, a girl who receives a single X chromosome containing the hemophilia gene can also have severe hemophilia. This is caused by a process called *non-random X chromosome inactivation*. Like all girls,

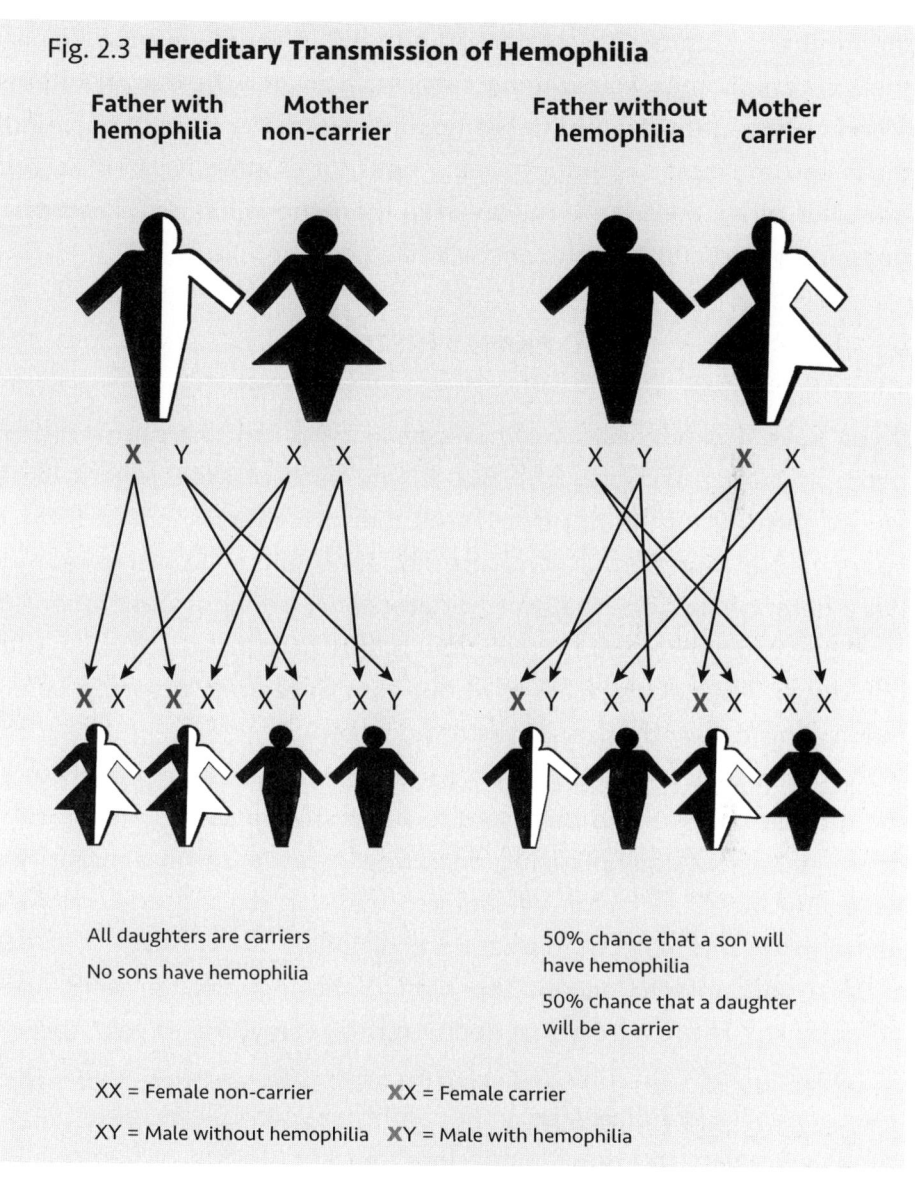

Fig. 2.3 **Hereditary Transmission of Hemophilia**

All daughters are carriers
No sons have hemophilia

50% chance that a son will have hemophilia
50% chance that a daughter will be a carrier

XX = Female non-carrier   XX = Female carrier
XY = Male without hemophilia XY = Male with hemophilia

she has two X chromosomes. Only one of these X chromosomes can be active, or functional, at a time—the second X chromosome is turned off or inactivated. This inactivation process is normally random: usually, one-half of the father's X chromosomes are turned off, and one-half of the mother's X chromosomes are turned off. In very rare instances, all the X chromosomes from one parent are inactivated. So if a girl inherits a hemophilia gene on the X chromosome from one parent, and all of the X chromosomes with functional genes for clotting factor inherited from the other parent are inactivated, then she will lack a functional gene for blood clotting, and she will have hemophilia.[8]

NO FAMILY HISTORY?

If you have a family history of hemophilia, you can test prenatally for hemophilia (see Chapter 13). But in one-third of cases, there is no known history of hemophilia, and the disorder is caused by a spontaneous mutation. This means that either the child or the mother has a hemophilia gene that was not present in previous generations.

How can you confirm that you're the first in your family with hemophilia? Speak to relatives about your ancestors, record a family medical history, and ask relatives to be tested.

When a child with hemophilia suddenly appears in the family tree, the mother may want to be tested to see if she's a carrier. Test results could influence family planning decisions. A carrier mother might also have low levels of factor VIII herself, may be diagnosed with mild hemophilia, and may bleed after trauma.

Are you able to accept the risks of having another child with hemophilia? That's a personal decision between you and your spouse or partner. Don't be influenced by pressure from your hematologist, your geneticist, medical labs, your neighbor, your in-laws, or inquiring minds who want to know! Increasing your knowledge of hemophilia, using this book and other sources, and adding your own real-life experiences will help you make the best family planning choices.

What Is Hemophilia?
Chapter 2 Summary

- Hemophilia is a rare genetic disorder that prevents blood from forming an effective clot.
- Hemophilia A occurs in approximately 1 in 5,000 male births.
- A child with hemophilia does not bleed faster, only longer.
- There are three basic stages in normal blood clotting: vasoconstriction, platelet plug, and fibrin clot.
- At least thirteen clotting factors in the blood work together in a specific sequence to form a fibrin clot.
- Hemophilia means that one of the clotting factors, usually factor VIII or factor IX, is missing or inactive.
- Your child can have severe, moderate, or mild hemophilia, depending on how much factor is active in his blood.
- Bleeds are controlled by infusions of clotting factor, called factor replacement therapy, or in the case of mild or moderate hemophilia, by desmopressin acetate.
- In one-third of cases, hemophilia occurs spontaneously with no family history.
- If the mother is a carrier, with each pregnancy she has a 50% chance of having a child affected by hemophilia (either having hemophilia or being a carrier).

∽ 3 ∽

The First Few Months

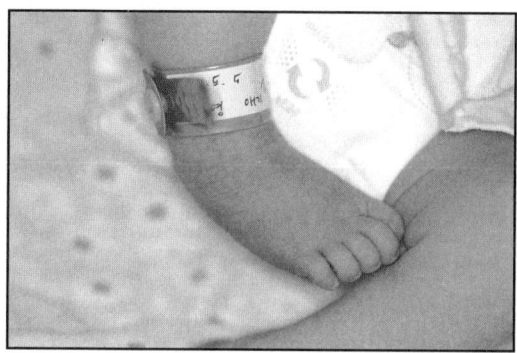

I was overwhelmed with the thought of caring for this precious bundle and didn't think I could get through the first months. My husband reminded me that we didn't have a choice—time to step up to the plate! So I began to focus on my child, not his bleeding disorder. Having hemophilia is only a small part of who he is. —Brendan Hayes, Texas

After the hemophilia diagnosis, your head may be spinning. You're juggling your feelings, coping with your family's reactions, caring for a new baby, and starting to learn about hemophilia. You must prepare for the unexpected, including possible bleeds in the first few months. You'll want to learn to recognize symptoms of various types of bleeds, while keeping in mind that some bleeds may never happen to your child. It just makes good parenting sense to know what can happen, how to avoid it, and how to take action if needed.

For many families, the first few months pass without a single incident or worry. But sometimes, these early months bring challenges. Three of the most common challenges are **circumcision**, vaccinations, and routine blood tests.

THE CIRCUMCISION DECISION

Circumcision is the surgical removal of the foreskin of the penis, an elective surgery often performed shortly after birth. Bleeding from circumcision is often the first indication that a child has a bleeding disorder, especially if hemophilia doesn't run in the family.

Can children with hemophilia be circumcised? Yes. Should they be? It's up to you. But if you know that hemophilia runs in your family, or you know you're having a child with hemophilia, you'll want to make an informed decision and prepare well before childbirth. First ask yourself why you want your child circumcised, and then weigh the risks, costs, and benefits.[1]

Circumcision is done for a variety of reasons, including medical, religious, cultural, and cosmetic. In the United States, the most common reason for circumcision is not medical but cosmetic—so a son will look like his father. The United States is the only country to suggest that the medical benefits of neonatal circumcision outweigh the risks. Medical organizations of all other countries agree that any medical benefits of circumcision do not outweigh the risks—in other words, there really is no compelling medical reason to have your child circumcised.[2]

The downside to circumcision? There are some medical risks:

- Prolonged bleeding, which varies depending on the method of circumcision used
- Infection (the risk is usually less than 1%, but up to 10% in some studies)
- Pain, if no anesthesia is used

Although anesthesia is used increasingly for circumcision, some physicians and some areas of the United States still don't use it routinely because it prolongs the procedure; and if the anesthetic is accidentally injected into a blood vessel of the penis, this can result in loss of the penis. *No baby should be circumcised without anesthesia.*

Circumcision without anesthesia is traumatic and causes severe pain.

Even if your child has hemophilia, a clot may form when minor bleeding occurs during circumcision. But that clot is not strong and may dislodge while your child is still in the hospital, or a week later when he's home. The resulting bleeding may color his diaper red, and this might surprise or shock you, though blood mixed with urine looks a lot worse than it is. On the other hand, arterial bleeding from a circumcision is serious, requiring treatment with factor and immediate emergency medical attention.

There are several different circumcision methods, and some have a lower risk of bleeding than others. Of the three most commonly used circumcision tools—the Mogen Clamp, the Gomco Clamp, and the Plastibell circumcision device—the Plastibell has the lowest risk of bleeding, but it's also associated with the highest risk of infection.

If you know your child has hemophilia and you want him circumcised, do your homework. *Don't feel pressured by anyone to have the circumcision immediately after birth*. First, contact your HTC to determine the type and severity of your child's disorder. Second, discuss in detail what the operation involves well before you give birth or agree to circumcision for your infant. Ask about these issues:

- Risks during and after the surgery
- Anesthesia during surgery and pain medication afterward
- The circumcision method to be used
- Care of the site
- Prolonged bleeding: Will your infant need his first infusion, or stitches?
- Costs, especially if factor is needed (many states don't provide **Medicaid** coverage for neonatal circumcision)
- Whether the surgery can be performed at your HTC

Several websites outline the risks of circumcision, and YouTube videos even show the operation. Speak to other parents of children with hemophilia to learn about their experiences. But don't feel pressured by friends, family, or your physician. An increasing number of American babies are uncircumcised, or intact. Only you, the parent, can decide if the medical or cultural benefits of circumcision outweigh the risks.

BLOOD TESTS AND IMMUNIZATIONS

Vaccinations are required for all infants. The chart on page 53 shows the recommended immunization schedule. Most vaccinations are administered by a needlestick, which may sometimes cause a bleed. Insist that your pediatrician administer vaccinations **subcutaneously** (under the skin), not in the muscles (an intramuscular injection). Subcutaneous injections have a much lower risk of bleeding compared to intramuscular injections.

If your child is suspected of having hemophilia, he will undergo diagnostic blood tests. Ask to have his umbilical cord blood drawn immediately after birth to perform some of these tests, and to avoid unnecessary needlesticks. Your child will also require additional sticks for further tests. Because it's sometimes hard to locate an infant's tiny veins, it may take a few tries to find a vein. And because babies don't always cooperate, medical staff may inadvertently hold your infant's arm too tightly while attempting to prevent it from moving while the needle is inserted. Staff may also apply a **tourniquet** too tightly (it takes less force to compress a child's veins than an adult's). All these actions may cause a bleed in the biceps or forearm. Bleeds like this are usually slow to appear, and you may see nothing for several hours to a day or more. Eventually, you might see black-and-blue marks or feel a hard lump in the muscle with no marks. If bruises (called **hematomas**) or lumps appear, apply ice and contact your HTC. Occasionally, a needlestick itself may also cause a bleed, with symptoms typically appearing within a few hours; these bleeds require factor treatment.

Circumcision: Religious Considerations

"My son Zack was circumcised by a *mohel* (medically certified rabbi) according to Jewish tradition, at our home. Following this religious ritual, before the rabbi left, he took great care to make sure Zack was doing well physically. Zack slept well that night, and didn't even wake up for a feeding. I thought he was just tired from the ordeal, but I awoke to find him in a blood-soaked diaper. I contacted the rabbi instead of going to the local emergency room, which my husband wanted to do. We went to the rabbi's home, and he told us that prolonged bleeding happens sometimes. He wasn't alarmed, and he quickly rewrapped the circumcision site with a sturdier bandage. He said he would take us to the local hospital if the bleeding didn't stop. The bleeding continued, and the rabbi cauterized the wound late that night. This finally stopped the bleeding. He even offered to have us stay at his home so he could monitor Zack's condition.

Almost 10 months later, Zack was finally diagnosed, and we had an explanation for all of his symptoms. I contacted the rabbi to inform him that Zack had severe hemophilia and to thank him again for his wonderful, compassionate care. He was surprised, and thought it was a miracle that he had been able to stop Zack's bleeding. It seems that **cauterization** doesn't work in all cases. He also said that he has circumcised boys with hemophilia! He just makes sure that they are infused first. I was shocked that he knew anything about hemophilia, but I later learned that in ancient times, rabbis documented bleeding after circumcision to establish family history.

My recommendation for Jewish families in the hemophilia community is to do some research before deciding to circumcise their sons. There are differences of opinion, depending on various interpretations of this religious act. But some well-informed rabbis can work with families and their doctors to perform a safe procedure while observing Jewish tradition. —Stephanie Dansker, California"

If you think your child has a muscle bleed, stay calm. This is usually not an emergency. Check the size of the affected area, and compare it to the other limb. Call your hematologist, who will probably recommend that you take your child to the emergency room or clinic for a dose of factor. If your child is in pain, ask what you can do to ease his discomfort.

> **Compartment Syndrome**
>
> Typical muscle bleeds are usually not emergencies. But in some cases, muscle bleeds can cause a serious complication called acute **compartment syndrome**, which is a medical emergency. Groups of organs or muscles, including their blood vessels and nerves, are organized into areas called compartments. Strong webs of connective tissue called **fascia** form the walls of these compartments, similar to insulation surrounding wires. During a muscle bleed, the muscle swells. There may also be bleeding into the compartment itself. The fascia of the compartment restricts the swelling, and pressure increases within the compartment. If the pressure is high enough, blood flow to the muscles in the compartment is restricted, starving muscles and nerves of oxygen and food. If the pressure in the compartment is not quickly reduced—usually by surgically opening up the compartment—then permanent nerve and muscle damage can result.

When it's time for immunizations or blood tests,

- Preferably, have vaccinations and blood tests done at an HTC.
- Request that vaccinations be administered subcutaneously.
- Apply pressure to the needlestick site for 10 minutes after a blood draw.
- If your child is on prophylaxis, schedule his doctor's appointment on the day you normally give factor.

- If your child is having blood drawn, ask that it be done by an experienced pediatric IV nurse or the person who is the "best stick" on duty.
- Hydrate your child well prior to blood draws (this helps keep the veins plump) and try to calm him during the procedure (because stress causes veins to constrict, staying calm helps keep them plump).
- If your son is having blood drawn, have the nurse apply dry heat to the IV area before the stick to raise the blood vessels.

With a little preparation, you'll sail through vaccinations and blood tests!

CHECK YOUR PREPAREDNESS LEVEL

After your child is born and you begin adjusting to the diagnosis, you usually have time to prepare for challenging situations. You read, surf the Web, look for families on Facebook, and speak to other parents and physicians. On the other hand, mastery of hemophilia comes only with experience. Prepare for things that might happen, and try to maintain perspective and humor. Think of hemophilia this way: although it's extremely unusual to be struck by lightning, you wouldn't stand under a tall tree during a thunderstorm. Similarly, not every type of bleed will happen to your child, but you should learn about their symptoms and treatment.

If your child is on prophy, you may not have to worry about many bleeds. If he isn't, the great news is that as he grows older and begins to talk and understand, he can tell you how he feels and where he hurts. You'll be able to respond quickly to his medical needs. Until then, read the next section on types of bleeds so you can prepare for possible scenarios.

TYPES OF BLEEDS

Because every child is unique, even children with the same factor deficiency and severity level experience bleeds in different ways. In other words, it's hard to give clear-cut answers or make predictions about *your* child's bleeding patterns. Remember that he will not bleed faster than someone without hemophilia—just longer.

Many things influence the way your child will bleed. But one thing is certain: considering his factor deficiency and severity level, he will be treated medically according to the type of bleed he experiences. There are usually three categories of bleeds:

- minor
- major
- severe

These categories are important because they help determine whether your child will receive factor, and they indicate the dose or amount of factor needed.

MINOR BLEEDS

Minor bleeds usually resolve quickly with a factor infusion, or may even stop bleeding on their own without factor. Minor bleeds can include early-onset muscle and joint bleeds, with no visible symptoms such as limping or stiffness.[3] Some minor bleeds can become major if not treated immediately. Here are some minor bleeds that probably won't require factor:

- scrapes
- bruises
- superficial cuts
- superficial mouth bleeds
- most nosebleeds

Use basic treatment for minor bleeds:

- First aid for cuts and scrapes: adhesive bandages and applied pressure
- Ice applied to a bruise
- Ice applied to the nose during a nosebleed
- Pinching the nose during a nosebleed
- Frozen Popsicles for most mouth bleeds[4]
- **Amicar** (aminocaproic acid) or Cyklokapron (tranexamic acid), called **antifibrinolytics**, for mouth bleeds and nosebleeds[5] after a factor infusion to help retain a clot

MAJOR BLEEDS

Major bleeds involve swelling and pain, and require one or more factor infusions. They include

- minor bleeds that don't stop bleeding on their own or need multiple factor infusions,
- muscle bleeds that limit motion, and
- joint bleeds (called **hemarthrosis**).

Minor bleeds become major bleeds when they don't stop on their own, even when you give a factor infusion. A bleed that seems inconsequential and not dangerous, like a toe bleed, can become dangerous if prolonged:

- Swelling can compress nerves and blood vessels or, if in the throat, can cut off the airway.
- Excessive blood loss can lead to **anemia** or low blood pressure and shock.

Bleeds in the mouth and throat are particularly troublesome:

- Superficial mouth bleeds are simply a nuisance, but bleeding in the tongue, floor of the mouth, cheek, or throat can cause swelling and make it hard to swallow or breathe.

- Blood can seep down inside the tissues of the neck, compressing the airway. This may happen slowly. If your child is recovering from a bleed in the tongue, cheek, floor of the mouth, neck, or throat, check periodically for swelling for a few days.

If your child has pain in the neck or throat, swelling, or trouble swallowing or breathing, then this is a medical emergency—you must take him to the hospital right away. All swelling in the neck or throat should be considered a bleed unless proven otherwise.

Your child will swallow some blood during mouth bleeds and nosebleeds. If he swallows a lot of blood, his stools will be black (not to be confused with dark-green stools, which are normal). Don't panic and assume it's an intestinal bleed. If his stools are black, check to see if he has a mouth bleed or nosebleed.

Muscle bleeds are hard to detect in young children and infants. Why? Because these bleeds aren't always visible and may show no bruising. If your child can't speak yet, he can't tell you that it hurts. The affected muscle may appear enlarged, have a lump, or be hard to the touch. Your child may avoid using the affected limb, or he may limp. Other signs and symptoms include a warm feeling in the muscle, enlarged veins, and numbness from pressure on nerves. If you're unsure about a muscle bleed in a limb, wrap a tape measure around the suspected area and compare its size to the opposite limb.

Muscle bleeds that cause compartment syndrome are always serious. If the muscle swells too much, it can put pressure on nerves and restrict the blood supply. This may cause permanent nerve and muscle damage and result in paralysis if the bleeding isn't stopped and the pressure rapidly reduced. Some muscle groups are large and, like sponges, can hold a lot of blood. These are serious bleeds. Always call your hematologist if you suspect a muscle bleed.

Joint bleeds usually happen in movable joints such as the elbow, knee, ankle, wrist, shoulder, hip, foot, or finger. These are the most common bleeds in people with hemophilia, comprising up to 80% of all bleeds.

3 The First Few Months

A joint is the space where two bones meet. Movable joints are surrounded by a tough fibrous joint capsule. Bleeding into a joint causes swelling within the capsule and, in severe cases, can cause the joint to temporarily lock in place. Children's joints are subject to a lot of movement. In children with severe hemophilia, jarring and pressure from normal running, jumping, and crawling can cause spontaneous bleeds (without apparent injury). Children with moderate and mild hemophilia typically get joint bleeds only after obvious injuries. But some children with moderate hemophilia may have spontaneous joint bleeds, just like children with severe hemophilia.

Here are some signs and symptoms[6] of a joint bleed:

- Swelling
- Reluctance to use the affected body part
- Limping, if the bleed is in the hips or lower extremities
- Warm, tingling sensation within the joint
- Extreme pain as bleeding continues
- Joint stiffness, or limited ability to extend or flex
- Keeping the limb in a slightly bent position to reduce pain and relieve pressure in the joint

Joint bleeds should be treated with factor immediately. A joint bleed is considered major when it results in limited use of a limb. Joint bleeds in certain areas of the body, such as the hip, are more dangerous than others and are considered severe.

Joint damage is the primary complication of hemophilia. Joint bleeds can cause joint damage. A single untreated bleed may cause permanent joint damage. Blood contains proteins, called **enzymes**, that digest or "eat" any blood that seeps outside the blood vessels. Enzymes help break down this escaped blood to speed its reabsorption into the body, which promotes healing. When bleeding occurs in a joint, enzymes also damage the cartilage—the smooth, glossy covering that protects the bone ends. This can make the joint stiff and painful. The result is a type of arthritis called **hemophilic**

arthropathy. In people with hemophilia, arthritis can happen even at a young age.

The sooner you treat a joint bleed, the sooner the bleeding stops, and the sooner your child can heal. Treat your child before stiffness, swelling, and limping occur, and you can help prevent early-onset arthritis. When in doubt, infuse. Never wait and see!

The great news is that with today's better products, prophy, and expert HTC care, we are raising a generation of children with little joint damage.

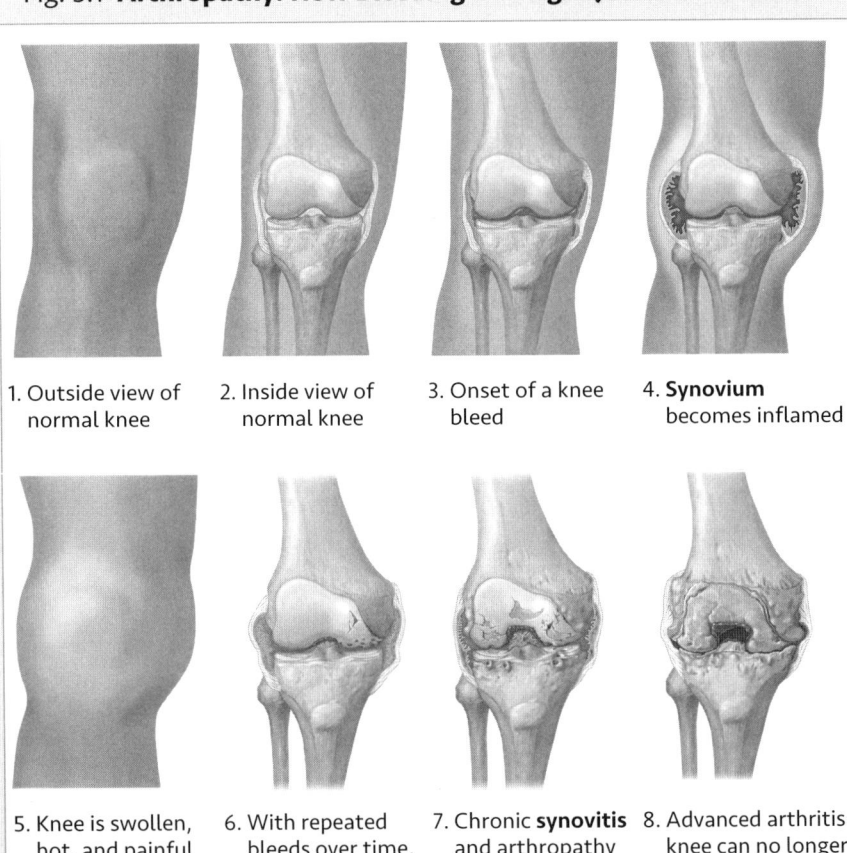

Fig. 3.1 **Arthropathy: How Bleeding Damages Joints Over Time**

1. Outside view of normal knee
2. Inside view of normal knee
3. Onset of a knee bleed
4. **Synovium** becomes inflamed
5. Knee is swollen, hot, and painful
6. With repeated bleeds over time, joint deteriorates
7. Chronic **synovitis** and arthropathy
8. Advanced arthritis: knee can no longer bend

Reprinted with permission. Illustrations by Robert Margulies, www.robertmargulies.com.

3 The First Few Months

SEVERE BLEEDS

This is probably the scariest part of the book—unless you consider the teenage years! But it's important to read about potentially serious bleeds, even if your child is on prophy and most of these bleeds will never happen. Severe bleeds are potentially life-threatening or can cause permanent nerve damage. But with prompt, correct treatment, there is little risk even if your child is not on prophy.

Severe bleeds include

- bleeds from surgery or dental work, and
- bleeds in the danger zones: muscle bleeds in the forearm, calf, groin, abdomen, or hip; bleeds in the throat, neck, or eye region; **gastrointestinal** (GI) tract bleeds; and head bleeds.

Bleeding during or after surgery that is not controlled with factor infusions is severe when it threatens recovery—and even the patient's life. Physicians will need to determine the cause of the bleeding, whether a blood vessel was damaged during surgery, or if a higher or more frequent dose of factor is needed. Bleeding from extensive dental work can be classified as severe when it seeps into the patient's throat and neck tissues, potentially closing off the airway.

Iliopsoas muscle bleeds (psoas) occur in the upper part of the thigh and into the groin, where the thigh muscle connects to the hip bone under the groin. Bleeding symptoms include pain in the hip, groin, stomach area, buttocks, or lower back. Your child may limp. He may not be able to stand up straight at the hip or be able to bend his leg to his chest while lying on his back. A lot of blood can be lost into the **iliopsoas** muscle compartment, causing acute compartment syndrome. Nerves that control leg movement pass through the iliopsoas muscle compartment. These nerves, as well as the muscles, can be cut off from their nourishing blood supply by the increasing pressure within the muscle compartment that results from a bleed. Treat these bleeds immediately, using factor doses around 100%, and consult your hematologist.

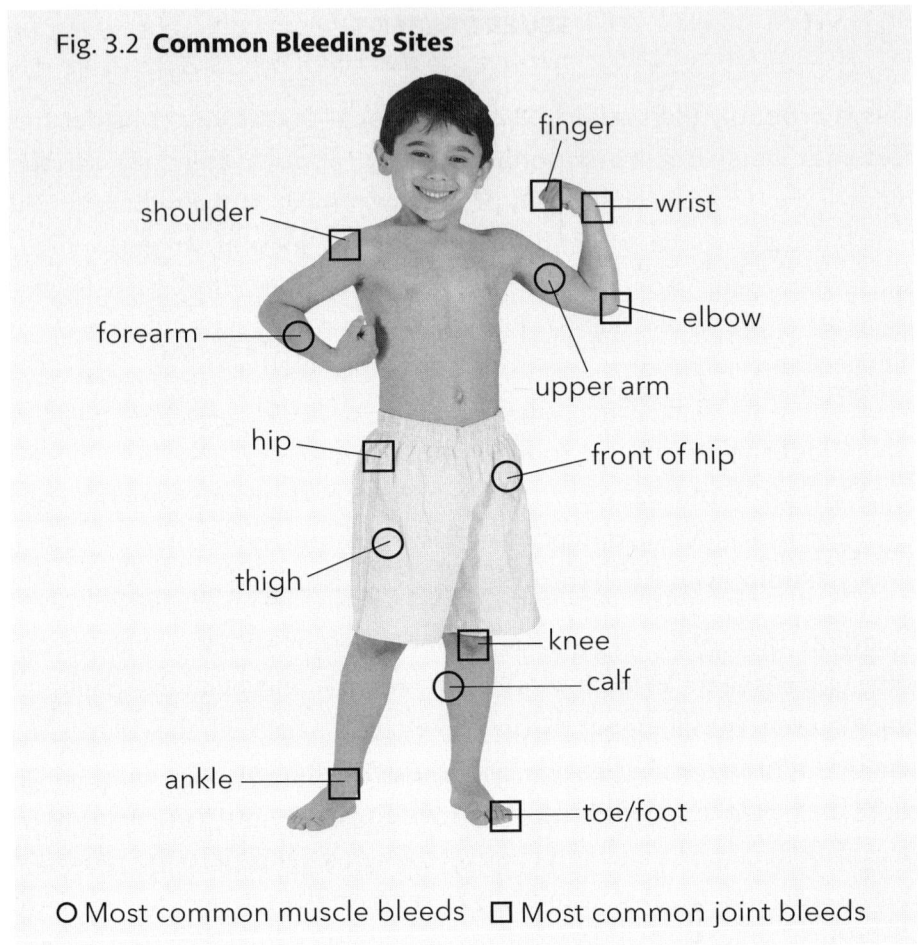

Fig. 3.2 **Common Bleeding Sites**

○ Most common muscle bleeds   ☐ Most common joint bleeds

Throat bleeds occur in the space at the back of the mouth, and can be hard to detect and easy to misidentify. Symptoms include swelling of the tissues inside the mouth or on the neck, choking, trouble swallowing, vomiting swallowed blood, and pain. These are dangerous bleeds because your child's airway, located in the throat, can be obstructed or even closed as a result of swelling caused by the bleed. If your child vomits blood but has no mouth bleed or nosebleed, have him examined immediately. If his tongue is swollen or bruised, look for extended swelling down the back of his throat. If your child gets tonsillitis or strep throat and coughs heavily for days, watch for signs of swelling or irritation of the throat. If you think he has the mumps, have him examined to rule out a throat bleed. Throat bleeds are very serious and should be treated immediately.[7] Always bring your child to the hospital if you suspect a throat bleed.

Neck bleeds are equally serious because they also can obstruct an airway. If your child seems to have a stiff or swollen neck or the mumps, call your hematologist immediately or bring your child to the ER for evaluation.

Eye bleeds are serious because of potential loss of eyesight due to pressure on the optic nerve. Also, eye sockets offer a pathway to the brain, where blood can seep. Report any pain, bruising, swelling, or black eyes to your hematologist.

Gastrointestinal bleeds happen in the stomach or intestines. Symptoms include coughing or vomiting blood, bloody stools (lower intestinal bleed) or black, tar-like stools (upper intestinal bleed), stomach pain, and swelling in the abdomen.

The digestive tract is rich with blood vessels; prolonged bleeding here can result in anemia or shock. These bleeds can be stopped only with factor. Injuries to the abdomen, some pain medications, and severe, prolonged coughing can sometimes cause GI bleeds. Call your hematologist immediately if you suspect this type of bleed.

Head injuries include any type of trauma to the head, from a bump—two children colliding on the playground—to serious concussions. Not every bump will cause a bleed. Head bleeds are hard to detect immediately, but fortunately, they are also uncommon. Your child should always wear a helmet while bike riding or participating in sports such as skiing or snowboarding. The symptoms of a head bleed can be similar to those of childhood viral diseases. Pooled blood presses on the brain and can interfere with sight, balance, and consciousness, and can cause vomiting and headaches. Assume that any significant bump to the head is a potential head bleed, and treat with factor; then consult your hematologist.

> **Symptoms of a Head Bleed**
>
> Call your hematologist *immediately* if your child has any of the following symptoms, especially if you know he has bumped his head:
>
> - neck stiffness
> - incessant crying
> - sensitivity to light
> - loss of consciousness
> - vomiting or projectile vomiting
> - lack of appetite
> - unequal pupil dilation
> - irritability
> - ear fluid leakage or dizziness
> - seizures
> - lethargy or sluggishness

Symptoms of a head bleed may not be obvious for several hours or even days after injury, and may not be accompanied by bruises or bumps. The blood can seep slowly and pool gradually. It's always risky to diagnose a head bleed by yourself when your child is an infant or toddler. Always call your hematologist. Together, discuss the injury and your child's reaction, and then monitor for symptoms of a bleed.[8] As your child gets older and becomes verbal, he can tell you how he feels, which helps in diagnosing a head bleed.

Don't be fooled by well-wishers, relatives in denial, know-it-alls, and people who are inexperienced with hemophilia—even doctors. They may tell you that the bleed is only on the "outside" if your child has a bump on his head, or that he isn't bleeding inside if he doesn't have a bruise. In truth, he could be bleeding both internally and externally, or he might not be bleeding at all. Always check with your HTC hematologist, even if it's just for your own peace of mind.

KEEP CALM AND CARRY ON

No one wants to imagine what it's like for an infant, toddler, or youngster to have a bleed. Don't stress yourself by imagining the

Recommended Childhood Immunization Schedule

Hib Vaccine
- First dose: 2 months
- Second dose: 4 months
- Third dose: 6 months
- Fourth dose: 12 to 15 months

Polio Vaccine
- First dose: 2 months
- Second dose: 4 months
- Third dose: 6 to 18 months
- Fourth dose: 4 to 6 years

DTaP Vaccine
- First dose: 2 months
- Second dose: 4 months
- Third dose: 6 months
- Fourth dose: 15 to 18 months
- Fifth dose: 4 to 6 years

Pneumococcal Vaccine
- First dose: 2 months
- Second dose: 4 months
- Third dose: 6 months
- Fourth dose: 12 to 18 months

MMR Vaccine
- First dose: 12 to 15 months
- Second dose: 4 to 6 years

Varicella Vaccine
- First dose: 12 to 18 months
- Second dose: 4 to 6 years

Hepatitis A (HAV) Vaccine
- Two doses at least 6 months apart. Recommended in selected areas for children over age 2. NHF Medical and Scientific Advisory Council (MASAC) Recommendation 151 advises that all children with hemophilia receive HAV vaccines.

Hepatitis B (HBV) Vaccine
- First dose: birth to 2 months
- Second dose: 1 to 4 months
- Third dose: 6 to 18 months
- After the initial series, booster shots are unnecessary. Can be given at any age, depending on the brand product and pediatrician recommendation. NHF MASAC Recommendation 151 advises that all children with hemophilia receive HBV vaccines.

Sources: www.medicinenet.com; www.cdc.gov; www.hemophilia.org

worst. Learn enough to be aware of possible bleeds, take the necessary precautions, and respond with appropriate actions. In almost all cases, prompt action—calling your hematologist, infusing with factor—will stop a bleed fast. Today, the emphasis is on preventing damage that results from incorrect or delayed therapy. You can treat quickly once you know what to look for.

It's hard to know how to diagnose bleeds and what to look for when your child is young and nonverbal. But don't worry! He'll soon be able to tell you what he feels and needs, making life with hemophilia much easier. In some ways, the first two years are the hardest, as you learn the ropes. In the coming years, you'll feel like you're gleefully swinging from those ropes. You'll find new freedom when your child can tell you he has a bleed. You'll have honed your skills and strengthened your hemophilia parent intuition. Until then, give yourself credit for all that you've learned and simply enjoy your baby, every day.

The First Few Months
Chapter 3 Summary

- Learn about types of bleeds so you'll be prepared. Most of them won't happen or will happen rarely, especially if your child is on prophylaxis.
- Make an informed decision about whether to circumcise your infant with hemophilia: learn the benefits and risks.
- Routine vaccinations and blood tests can cause muscle bleeds.
- Have your pediatrician give subcutaneous vaccinations, not in the muscle.
- Minor bleeds may not require factor.
- Major bleeds cause swelling and pain and always require factor.
- Severe bleeds can cause permanent damage or happen in areas of the body that make them life-threatening.
- Bleeding into joints damages cartilage, eventually causing permanent joint damage.
- When in doubt, infuse. Treat aggressively.

4

The Doctor-Parent Partnership

I have the right to be an equal partner in determining the best treatment for my son. I have the right to be heard and listened to. Not only do many healthcare professionals have little firsthand experience with bleeding disorders, none of them knows my son the way I do. Fortunately, many physicians welcome our input, especially when we are respectful and show that we are knowledgeable. —Ann-Grete Tan, Pennsylvania

The hemophilia community is fortunate to have access to specialized, competent, dedicated, compassionate doctors, nurses, and other medical staff. You'll meet these professionals at your HTC. They are experienced with hemophilia, know the right questions to ask, and can give you the care and information you need. Many parents develop a close relationship with their HTC staff and often refer to them as friends and even family.

Your experience in an emergency room (ER) may be a different story! Attempting to get help at an ER, especially during your first few visits, may seem like an exercise in frustration. After all, hemophilia is rare, and most doctors don't meet people with hemophilia regularly, if ever. Although most small ERs are not as hectic as portrayed on television, ER physicians have a huge spectrum of cases to diagnose and treat. If they're unaware of hemophilia's complications and your child appears to be healthy, they may not rank hemophilia as high in urgency as gunshot wounds, drug overdoses, car wrecks, or poison ingestion.

You may have to educate and even challenge a doctor who is unfamiliar with hemophilia. This isn't always easy. For some parents, challenging authority figures is difficult. Doctors, with their many years of schooling and specialized knowledge, can seem intimidating. Hospitals, with their twisting corridors, strange smells, and rigid rules, can be overwhelming. Initially, it's a relief to hand over much of your decision-making power to doctors because you are so dependent on them. But as your child's advocate, you must soon take a proactive role in healthcare decisions to ensure a positive treatment outcome.

MEDICAL PERSONNEL YOU'LL MEET

An HTC guarantees the best care for your child. HTCs offer **comprehensive care**: specialists in hemophilia who attend to every health aspect, including medical, social, dental, physiological, and nutritional needs.

Who will you meet at the HTC? What role will each person play in your child's care?

Hematologist: a specialist in treating blood disorders. Your assigned hematologist will see your child at least once or twice a year to monitor his development and test his blood.[1]

Nurse coordinator: works with the hematologist. As the person you'll see most often, the nurse coordinator offers educational materials, interviews you, and performs infusions in the clinic. In an HTC, he or she is often the hemophilia clinic coordinator.

Pediatrician: your child's regular physician, who specializes in infant and child development. Your pediatrician should defer all hemophilia-related questions and treatments to the HTC, while continuing to handle all routine baby questions, immunizations, and illnesses. The pediatrician also monitors normal development. Because these doctors aren't necessarily part of an HTC, you may want to keep the pediatrician you saw before you learned of your child's hemophilia.

Social worker: helps parents cope when raising a child with medical problems by offering a listening ear and coping strategies. Your social worker can provide advice and resources regarding financial aid, insurance, and social support groups. As your child grows into adolescence, your social worker will counsel your child directly about school, personal responsibilities, and health.

When necessary, your hematologist or nurse coordinator may refer you to these specialists:

Orthopedist: a specialist in bone and joint development and injuries. An orthopedist may occasionally examine your child's joints for signs of damage following bleeds or at the yearly checkup. In addition to surgery, this specialist can also provide protective and corrective devices, such as casts and splints, to aid healing in joints and bones.

Physical therapist: a specialist in muscle development and motor coordination. The physical therapist can help guide your child's rehabilitation after an injury and suggest safe activities to help strengthen muscles that protect joints.

Geneticist: a specialist in genetic disorders. The primary job of a geneticist is determining whether any females in the family are carriers of the hemophilia gene. The geneticist can also offer genetic counseling for families considering having more children.

Radiologist: a specialist in noninvasive diagnostic techniques for viewing and analyzing internal organs and tissues. These techniques include x-ray, magnetic resonance imaging (MRI), **computed tomography** (CT) scan, **ultrasound**, and positron emission tomography (PET) scans. Some of these procedures can detect internal bleeding, such as **intracranial hemorrhage** (ICH), before signs or symptoms appear.

Laboratory technician: may draw blood from your child. The lab tech performs laboratory tests that help your physician determine whether your child has hemophilia; the type of factor deficiency and level of severity; and evidence of a blood-transmitted infection.

The following doctors may be part of the ER team that can treat your child in an emergency, or when injuries occur after normal working hours and the regular hematology clinic is closed:

ER attending physician: a specialist in emergency care who may be the first to examine your child. This doctor might be an intern, resident, or full-time physician. Interns are first-year postgraduate physicians training in residency. Residents are upper-level postgraduate physicians, usually in their second through fifth year of training. ER attending physicians may know some, a little, or nothing about treating a child with hemophilia. Interns and residents should coordinate with the hematologist-on-call when treating your child.[2]

Hematologist-on-call: the hematologist for emergencies. During regular working hours, you can see your nurse coordinator or hematologist in the clinic if you have an emergency. All the hematologists in the HTC rotate shifts, so on weekends you may reach your own hematologist as the hematologist-on-call, if it's a nonemergency. If you reach other hematologists at the same hospital, they may not know much about hemophilia if they aren't part of the HTC staff. Remember that most hematologists specialize in oncology (the study and treatment of cancer), and not bleeding disorders.

Familiarize yourself with the titles and responsibilities of all specialists who might see your child. Then you'll know to request an orthopedist if your child has recurring trouble with his ankles. During a middle-of-the-night emergency, when the ER attending physician's answers haven't satisfied you, you'll know to request the hematologist-on-call.

YOUR RIGHTS AND RESPONSIBILITIES IN THE HOSPITAL

As a parent, you are the main advocate for your child. You protect and defend your child's best interests, and you speak out on his behalf. You know your child better than anyone does, and it's your job to protect him from unnecessary physical and emotional harm. But in a medical setting, you may lack confidence when doctors and nurses test, prick, and prod him, and when you know little about hemophilia.

4 The Doctor-Parent Partnership

To be a good advocate for your child, realize that you have rights. In most cases, these rights aren't written as law. But they can be defended by law, and they are your rights as your child's advocate and a customer of the hospital. That's correct: you are a customer, and the hospital is a business. In the field of economics, "Hospitals" come just before "Hotels" in the United States list of service sectors, and the comparisons are obvious. You are hiring this business to serve you, and you have many of the same rights as when dealing with any service provider—competent staff, prompt service, and knowing what you pay for.

Most physicians know and respect these rights. But occasionally, your rights may be ignored, particularly in times of crisis or when medical staff is unfamiliar with hemophilia. Advocating for your child helps you feel more involved and capable. Advocating becomes easier when you know your rights, because then you can exercise them.

YOUR RIGHTS AS A PARENT

Parents should take an aggressive role in their child's treatment. Question every treatment to determine if it is desirable for someone with a bleeding disorder. Don't be scared to stand up and ask questions or voice your opinion. It's worth it. —Micki Fields, Oklahoma

You have the right to stay with your child. This is the simplest and easiest way to help. You can hold your child, whisper to him, distract him during procedures, stroke his head, and let him know you're there. But stay calm. If you become visibly disturbed or angry, you'll upset your child and hinder the medical staff.

You may want to stay with your child to ensure that procedures are followed correctly. You might know the easiest veins for venipuncture or the way your child prefers to be held. Some staff may not know the best approach, and may even try something that isn't appropriate for hemophilia, such as accessing a neck vein for drawing blood or for infusing factor, or delaying factor treatment until an x-ray is performed.

You have the right to refuse treatment, procedures, or drugs if your child is not in a life-threatening situation. You can postpone diagnostic tests and procedures such as x-rays and request that your child be infused first. You can refuse additional blood tests that you deem unnecessary for the moment, such as **carrier tests** for you. First, be sure you're making an informed decision: talk to your physician about the appropriateness and usefulness of the test. Your medical team may override this right if your child's life is in danger.

You have the right to prompt treatment. Children with hemophilia should be examined as quickly as possible, particularly after head, neck, or joint injuries. Unfortunately, not every hospital understands this, and the staff may not see visible proof that your child needs immediate treatment. Explain what happened, what's going on inside your child's body, and why he needs prompt treatment. Be assertive and specific: "I need to be seen in fifteen minutes." To support your demand to be seen immediately, it helps to carry a letter from your hematologist (see Appendix C) containing information about emergency care for your child and phone numbers of your HTC staff.

You have the right to be treated respectfully and courteously. Most parents have great relationships with their medical team. But as in any profession, you'll meet some arrogant, unreasonable medical staff. You can always report rudeness or insensitivity to a staff member's superiors, and you can tell the person directly that insensitive or unprofessional behavior or comments are unacceptable.

You have the right to change physicians or ask for another ER physician. If you believe the attending physician isn't listening to you or is not following correct procedure for an infusion, you can request another physician or the head of the ER. You can also call your hematologist for support. Listen to your parental instincts.

If you have an ongoing problem in your relationship with your regular hematologist, consider changing doctors, even if it means getting another doctor in the same practice.

You have the right to request an infusion of factor for your child. If your child has a bleed and staff discourages or refuses an infusion, ask why. If you don't get a reasonable answer, and you are certain that the injury needs factor treatment, insist on an infusion. If you still meet resistance, have the attending physician document on paper that he or she refused to give your child an infusion. This could have important repercussions later if your child suffers from not being infused and you need to settle the outcome in court.

You have the right to have treatments, medicine, and procedures explained to you before they are done. When a nurse or physician orders a procedure, such as a blood test, CT scan, or MRI, ask why the procedure is necessary and how it will be done. Ask how the test results will change your child's treatment. For example, a physician may order a CT scan following a minor head bump, yet studies have shown that CT scans miss 95% of early head bleeds. Does a negative CT scan mean that you shouldn't treat for a possible bleed? No! A suspected head bleed should always be treated. Staff must adequately answer your questions before you consent to treatment. Ask your medical staff these questions:

- What are the possible side effects?
- What medicine and dosage will be given?
- Will the procedure hurt my child?
- What should the results be?[3]

You have the right to get someone else to do the venipuncture. Many parents set a limit of two or three attempts by one medical staff person to secure a vein. If no vein is secured, parents will intervene and request another staff member. This method eliminates the person's increasing stress when unable to get a vein, and offers a new person a fresh chance, possibly protecting your child's veins from wear and tear. Your anxiety is reduced—and so is your child's.

You have the right to tell medical staff about your medical situation and personal policies, and to be respected. You probably know how the injury occurred and how your child reacted. You may know more about the infusion procedure. You know the best veins to try and how much factor your child should receive. You may want your hematologist to call the ER before your visit. Always tell medical staff what you know, bring literature to prove it, and admit what you don't know.

You have the right to see your child's medical records at your request, if your child is younger than 18. This right is defended by law, and any request to see these records must be honored.

You have the right to have all consent forms explained to you before signing. It's hard to read consent forms in the middle of an ER, with your child in pain. But try to read them, or at least ask what you are signing. You may not agree with everything you sign, and until you become familiar with the operations of your particular hospital, you should question everything.

You have the right to know of any research studies being conducted on your child. Your physician may ask if you're interested in participating in new product testing or studies on hemophilia patients. You don't have to participate; but researchers are trying to improve care for children with hemophilia, and they need critical information about treatment. If you'd like to help, get as much information as possible about the study before agreeing.

You have the right to private explanations, without your child or other patients present. Sometimes doctors overload new parents with information about their child or the diagnosis—in the waiting room, with other parents and patients. This violates your right to privacy, forces you to handle your emotions in public, and distracts you from absorbing information. If doctors give you information in an inappropriate location, simply ask them to find a private room where you can confer.

We've reviewed some of your basic rights. Now it's up to you to make sure they are respected. At times, you'll need to ask to have things done your way. If you're not naturally assertive, you'll have to learn. Practice these statements and questions:

- What needle size are you using for the infusion? Can you please use a 25-gauge needle?[4]
- May we go somewhere private to discuss this first?
- I allow only three needlesticks per medical staff person. Could I please have another staff member?
- I need to stay with my child to comfort him. I won't hinder the procedure.
- We were taught to infuse first, x-ray later.
- Have you ever treated a child with hemophilia before?

YOUR RESPONSIBILITIES AS A PARENT

If you want doctors to respect your rights, you must show that you are responsible. Here are some guidelines to follow:

Give medical staff the correct and complete information. What is your child's factor deficiency and level? Which product do you use? What is its brand name and unit size? What are the facts of the injury? Are your child's immunizations up to date?

Treat healthcare professionals with respect and courtesy. Stick to the issue at hand, and don't turn the visit into a personal confrontation. Never call people names, use foul language, or yell. Remember that you need the help of the ER staff.

Respect hospital rules and regulations, and follow them when they make sense. Of course, there are exceptions to every rule. Although you want the hospital to meet your specific needs, try to adapt your needs to meet the hospital's huge patient caseload. If you feel uneasy, ask questions about treatment plans, procedures, and tests preferably before they are carried out. See if the explanations make sense to you—sometimes the nurse or technician performing the tests may not be able to explain clearly. If an explanation doesn't make sense, don't feel obliged to follow the rules.

Contact the Patient Relations office. Speak to a hospital mediator when there is a problem you can't resolve with medical staff.

Show the staff that you are a responsible and assertive parent. Try to behave calmly and firmly. This will help you earn respect. Be prepared to assist, and remember that this is a team effort with your child's health as the common goal. Because problems can sometimes turn into personal conflicts, with parents and staff blaming each other, you must focus on the medical issue, not on the doctor or nurse, while keeping in mind the outcome you want.

> Keep scheduled appointments, or call in advance to cancel or reschedule. The HTC may call you annually to help you keep your clinic visit, but you are responsible for keeping your child healthy by making regular visits. At the very least, visit your HTC annually!

YOUR RIGHT AND RESPONSIBILITY TO QUESTION

Even after receiving factor for a tongue bleed, Evan was still bleeding. My nurse coordinator suggested I go to the ER and get a second infusion and possibly a suture. I waited over two hours in the ER, and I finally demanded to see the doctor. He examined Evan and told me to take him home, that I was overly concerned. I said, "I'm supposed to get more factor; I just wanted your opinion as to whether he should get a suture." I was told again that Evan would be fine. Meanwhile, Evan was crying and spitting up blood. I politely asked if the doctor had read Evan's charts and knew that he had severe hemophilia. The doctor hesitated and then glared at me, saying, "Are you questioning my judgment?" I said, "I most definitely am! I know how my child responds to treatment, and he's not responding well." The doctor left the room and canceled the order for more factor. I was so frustrated and exhausted that I waited until the next morning to have Evan treated at our HTC.

—Kris Boehmer, Michigan

Questioning medical decisions and procedures is a right *and* a responsibility. You have the right to learn what, why, and how. You have the responsibility to protect your child. When you ask questions, you'll . . .

- learn more about medical procedures and risks,
- become more independent,
- catch mistakes before they're made, and
- develop the confidence to challenge a doctor's orders when you think something isn't right.

Some medical decisions are based on general policy or legal protection, and others are made for your child's immediate health and safety. Ask why any test or procedure has or has not been ordered. Ask about the risks if you refuse to allow the procedure.

You may also question why a doctor chooses not to infuse your child. This is rare because most doctors err on the side of safety. If your instinct says to infuse, then insist on it. Remember: When in doubt, infuse.

WHAT DOCTORS SHOULD KNOW

Most HTC physicians deal superbly with parents and families. They are concerned, devoted, and approachable. But there are many kinds of people, and many kinds of doctors. You may meet a doctor who appears insensitive to you or your child's emotional and physical needs. Or one who challenges your confidence and intimidates you. Stand your ground, and ask to be treated fairly.

If you're a healthcare provider who treats hemophilia patients, use the following advice, gleaned from more than 160 parents who agree that effective and professional medical personnel should follow these guidelines:

Listen to parents. When parents tell you their child needs to be infused, he does. If parents say that the infusion is easier with their child sitting on a lap, trust their judgment.

Be patient with parents. Like you, parents are under stress. Protective parental instinct is strong when a child is in pain and needs medical treatment. Parents may question, argue, or cry.

Don't overload parents with information. Give them time to absorb things. Talk to parents privately, and make sure they understand. "It's after the physician leaves that the questions and concerns start popping up," shares one mom.

Talk to the child and siblings directly when possible. Children with hemophilia will someday be responsible for their own care. If they have a role in making decisions, they will be ready to take over at an appropriate age. If brothers and sisters also understand the process, they can be more helpful to their sibling.

Be direct with the parents. They can handle it, even if they need a good cry first. Parents have the right to know why treatments are delayed or aren't working.

Rely on parents' judgment. This applies particularly to doctors who aren't hematologists. Don't second-guess a parent who recommends dosage or treatment or describes the extent of an injury.

Respond politely to parents' questions. Parents have a right to know why certain tests are ordered and certain decisions made. Encourage them to offer their advice as experienced parents.

Let parents participate in procedures as much as possible. When parents show that they are responsible and calm, allowing them a sense of control can reduce their stress level.

Admit when you do not know how to diagnose a hemophilic bleed. Consult with someone more experienced. Parents don't expect you to know everything, but they do expect sound judgment.

No more than three needlesticks. Please don't subject children to pain because you want to complete the infusion yourself. Never use the **jugular vein** or femoral vein.[5]

Give the infusion your full attention. Have all medical supplies ready, the correct needle size, and factor mixed. Don't undertake unnecessary procedures; for example, you don't need an IV drip for an infusion.

Do not attempt to make parents feel guilty. Never blame parents for their child's injury or for having children with hemophilia. Never act discouraged, and never use negative language in front of a child.

When in doubt, infuse! Don't discount the pain or symptoms of a child with hemophilia. Ignoring or misreading symptoms can result in severe or long-term damage.

EFFECTIVE EMERGENCY ROOM VISITS

As a parent, you may visit the emergency room frequently during the first few months or even years after your child is born. You'll go there when your HTC is closed, usually at night or on weekends, or when you have an emergency.

Even if you initially spend many nights or weekend days at the ER, please don't think your life will always be like this. Soon life will get back to normal, and you'll be happily complaining about the time you spend at Little League, piano lessons, soccer practice, and the orthodontist!

Why do you need to visit the ER so often when your child is first diagnosed? The main reason is that you are inexperienced at detecting bleeds or giving your child factor. You go to seek advice or have someone give a needlestick. As your child grows, and as you learn to infuse him yourself, you'll visit the ER less often.

Make ER visits more bearable and productive. Know what to expect beforehand, so you don't feel so lost, disempowered, or emotional. When you're prepared, you'll feel ready to handle almost anything.

THE EMERGENCY ROOM SYSTEM

ER physicians screen patients based on the perceived urgency of their medical condition—not on a first-come, first-served basis. The process of registering, sorting, and prioritizing patients is called **triage**.

When you arrive at the ER, you'll enter the waiting area and meet with the triage nurse. The triage nurse prioritizes when your child will be seen, so make sure you stress the urgency of the need for medical care. In addition to making a triage assessment, the nurse will record on an admittance sheet your child's name, the diagnosis of hemophilia, and a description of the injury. The triage nurse will also ask if your child has allergies to any medications and whether his inoculations are current. Your child may get a hospital band for his wrist, printed with his name and the date. You may need to fill out an insurance form or see an admitting processor, who will probably check information for accuracy: your pediatrician's name, your insurance company and home address, and your child's birthdate.

If you use the ER in your local hospital, not in an HTC, it's best to have a **protocol** in place before you visit. Ask your HTC staff to provide in-service training to educate your local ER staff. Provide phone numbers to keep the lines of communication open. Don't wait for the first emergency visit to educate your local hospital staff. Planning and teamwork will help ensure that they can provide appropriate care.

The admittance sheet goes with you to an examination room, which may be a private room or a large room with screened partitions, where you may be asked to remove your child's clothes. A nurse or doctor will examine him with a stethoscope and take his blood pressure, and then weigh him in order to calculate his factor dosage. The rest of the exam—perhaps checking eyes, ears, abdomen—will assure staff that there are no other complications. A blood pressure reading is important: after the infusion, your child's blood pressure may be taken again to note any changes, in case he has a reaction to the factor.

After this exam, you may be asked to return to the waiting room.

The wait may be long, so bring supplies with you: diapers, toys, juice or formula, snacks. Fridays and Saturdays are usually more crowded, and the waits are longer.

When you are called, you'll be sent to a treatment room, which may or may not be private. You'll wait here until a doctor arrives. The doctor will ask about your child, probably repeating questions already asked: What kind of hemophilia does he have? How did the injury take place? Is he allergic to medicines? Has he had all his immunizations? The doctor may examine your child's ears, eyes, and abdomen. If your child has a head injury, the doctor may spend a lot of time checking pupil reactions and looking for fluid in the ear, which could indicate serious damage. These exams don't hurt your child, but especially if he is under three, he will probably cry. His injury may be painful; he may be afraid of having a stranger touch him; or he may be uncomfortable in a strange environment.

The doctor may appear to delay treatment, asking questions that don't seem relevant to the problem itself: When did you first learn your child has hemophilia? When did he get his first bleed? Or after examining your child, the doctor may disappear for a long time, perhaps twenty minutes. The doctor is probably checking hospital records or conferring with specialists. If it feels too long to you, ask another doctor or nurse, directly but politely, what is causing the delay. Keep reminding them of your needs.

After your child has been examined, and you and the doctor together decide that he needs an infusion, the doctor will order factor from the hospital if you didn't bring your own.[6] Your child will be infused. After the infusion, the doctor will want to see if your child has a reaction to the factor and perhaps briefly examine him again. If your child has a severe joint injury or any kind of suspected or actual head injury, the doctor may request an x-ray or CT scan. Unfortunately, this will involve more waiting.

Parents report that the first few ER trips are usually long and frustrating, unless the ER is not crowded. Expect to spend several hours on your initial visits until you learn the ropes.

DON'T LEARN THE HARD WAY: PREPARE FOR YOUR ER VISIT

You can learn to make the ER experience more effective and positive, but don't learn through trial and error. Take advantage of the experiences of many parents before you, who share their wisdom here. Parents usually zero in on two challenges at the ER:

- Unnecessarily long waits
- Physicians who are inexperienced with hemophilia

Here's how to navigate the ER to make the system work for you:

- Before you go to the ER, phone the hematologist-on-call, if possible, to discuss your child's injury, symptoms, and treatment.
- Ask the hematologist-on-call to alert ER staff and get your child's records.
- If your hospital doesn't have a hematologist-on-call, call the ER directly and tell the staff to expect you.
- Bring factor with you if you store it at home.[7]
- When you arrive, give the triage nurse all your updated information, including allergies, immunization dates, insurance carrier, and insurance changes.
- Tell the triage nurse how urgently your child the needs to be examined.
- Make sure the nurse writes everything down! Sometimes a triage nurse neglects to write "hemophilia" on the form. The doctor will read only "knee injury," and your child may be placed low on the priority list.

If you have to wait an hour when your child has a head injury, joint injury with swelling and pain, or bleeding into the abdomen, you have waited too long. Go to the triage nurse and demand—really demand—that your child be seen quickly. Show the nurse his medical ID with "hemophilia" inscribed on it. Show a letter from his physician, an article on emergency hemophilia care, or this book. Raise a ruckus, get a little crazy, but get their attention!

4 The Doctor-Parent Partnership

Once you make it to the treatment room, you may face further delays. Some doctors, inexperienced with hemophilia, will ask you a series of questions unrelated to the current injury. You may feel frustrated. You've had a long drive with an injured, cranky child and waited a long time in a crowded ER. Doctors ask these questions because they so rarely see children with hemophilia, and they may use this opportunity to learn more. Tell the doctor that you'll gladly answer general questions later, but your child needs to be infused immediately.

Record your child's name in the ER log, if one is available. This log contains information about his hemophilia and treatment. In the future, if a doctor doesn't listen to you or questions your knowledge, refer the doctor to your child's name and medical information in the log.

When the infusion is over, the attending physician may want to observe your child for reactions. Be prepared for a wait!

Parents of children with hemophilia are tenacious. "Never underestimate the power of a hemophilia mother!" writes one. Some doctors haven't encountered parents like them before. Although ER staff members handle all kinds of accidents, injuries, and illnesses, hemophilia may be something new. To receive fast, satisfactory care, you must be well informed about hemophilia, and well informed about your child's injuries and treatment preferences. In time, you'll train your doctors to trust you, listen to you, and respond to you. And in turn, you'll also come to appreciate and understand their schedules, commitments, and professional responsibilities. Together, you'll meet in the middle, where respect and responsibility thrive, for the sake of our children with hemophilia.

The Doctor-Parent Partnership
Chapter 4 Summary

- To protect your child, ensure a positive treatment outcome, and maintain control of situations, you must be part of the medical decision making.
- HTCs offer comprehensive care: hemophilia specialists attend to social, dental, physiological, nutritional, and treatment needs.
- Learn the titles and functions of the medical staff caring for your child at the HTC and ER. You'll be able to request a specialist when needed.
- You have specific rights as a parent. When you know your rights, you can exercise them in a medical setting. You have the right to be heard and treated promptly and respectfully.
- You have responsibilities as a parent. These include sharing all information with your medical team and being respectful. Work as a team with your medical staff.
- Initially, you might spend a lot of time at the ER. When you learn more about hemophilia and start infusing your child yourself, you'll make far fewer trips to the ER.
- To shorten long waits:
    Learn about hemophilia.
    Know ER procedures.
    Call ahead.
    Bring your own factor.
    Question procedures.
    Voice your needs.

5

The First Year

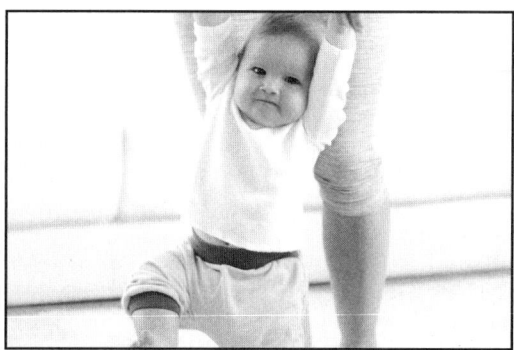

Our doctor explained that the first year would be the "honeymoon." She said chances were that our child wouldn't experience a bleed. Six hours later, we were back in that ER with that same doctor treating a bleed in his right elbow from the venipuncture she did to determine his factor level! —Anonymous

The first year of a baby's life is filled with joyful firsts: first smile, first teeth, first steps, first birthday. If this is your first baby, the firsts are even more special. All babies reach unique milestones to record and remember. But your baby's list of firsts may include the first signs of hemophilia—and perhaps the first infusion of factor.

It's an anxious time, adjusting to life with hemophilia. You may be waiting and wondering when the first bleed or infusion will occur. How will it happen? Will you hold yourself together emotionally?

You can reduce your anxiety by being prepared. This chapter will show you how to

- familiarize yourself with normal child developmental milestones,
- learn how your baby's development can naturally lead to bleeds,
- avoid unnecessary injuries,
- speed up the healing process when injuries do occur, and
- maintain a greater sense of emotional control.

When you feel prepared and confident, you can relax and enjoy your baby's amazing first year of growth, exploration, socialization, and achievement.

OUR LITTLE "BRUISERS"

Bruises happen when blood seeps into the tissue surrounding a torn blood vessel. They are probably the most common sign of hemophilia in babies and young children. Because of this, parents can become overly concerned with each little bruise. Although bruises in children with hemophilia are a bit more colorful, they're rarely serious.

Bruises may look unsightly—and just plain wrong on a baby. But expect to see bruising, and expect people to look at you curiously. Strangers may ask you questions in an accusing tone. You can reply with facts about hemophilia, or you can just say thanks, and tell the questioner that your child is extremely active. Remember, you are now an empowered parent! You can choose who to inform and how to inform.

Bruising is a normal part of your child's development. So is being held affectionately by his parents. Yet you may find that even holding your child in a certain way, or picking him up, can leave small bruises. But don't let bruises stop you! Always pick up and hold your child without worrying.

Bruising often makes a dramatic debut around age five months if your child uses a walker. Most pediatricians in the United States advise against using walkers because of the sudden mobility they give infants—and the increased danger of serious injury from falls. If your child uses a walker, bruises may appear on his ribcage and chest, where he thrusts against the walker. They may also appear on his thighs, where his legs rest on the seat. These bruises can be large, in shades of red and black, but they're usually harmless. They may take a long time to heal, aggravated by continued use of the walker. You can minimize this problem by padding the walker.[1]

When bruises blossom, apply ice to relieve pain and prevent further bruising, if your infant or toddler will let you.[2] Make a note of the bruise and how your child is reacting. Use a pen to draw an outline around the bruise on his skin. If the bruise spreads beyond this marked boundary, you may want to call your HTC for reassurance.

You can tell that a bruise is healing by its color and size. On light-colored skin, a fresh bruise, especially near the surface, usually looks red because of blood leaking into the tissues (deep bruises may skip this step). Within a few hours, the blood leaking from the injured blood vessel loses oxygen, turning the bruise blue or purple. Dark red anywhere on a bruise is a sign of renewed bleeding under the skin. As the blood is broken down over the next one to three days, the bruise turns from purple to blackish-blue. When the bruise begins to heal during the next two to four weeks, it will turn greenish, then yellow. Yellow means that the blood is almost reabsorbed. You may notice a large white bump in the center of a bruise. This means that the bruising is deep in the skin. Bruises are harder to identify on dark-colored skin. Fortunately, the tendency to bruise lessens as a child matures and develops muscles and greater coordination.

TEETHING

Infants usually start teething at age three to seven months. The mouth becomes the center of their universe, and they actively seek out objects to suck on. Babies sometimes teethe on sharp or hard items that can cause mouth bleeds. Mouth bleeds can result from a small cut on the gums, a nip on the tongue, a tear in the **frenulum** (the skin that attaches the upper lip to the gums), or the eruption of new teeth. Mouth bleeds are tricky to treat. You can't apply a bandage, you can't apply pressure, and the injury can't dry up because babies seem to have an infinite capacity to drool. Although every child experiences teething, many infants with hemophilia have no teething bleeds.

Mouth bleeds can be messy and may take a long time to heal. Instead of dripping clear infant drool, your child will drip red drool. You'll want to use bibs and wash his sheets and shirts more often.

A mouth bleed might be your child's first bleed and your first sight of his blood. If you're surprised, shocked, or scared, just remember that it almost always looks worse than it is. Blood mixed with saliva looks like more blood than is really there.

But you'll still want to be sure your child is okay. Check his mouth when he has a bleed, and determine the origin. Did he cut his mouth, is a new tooth coming in, or did he suck on a red felt-tipped pen? If the blood is dripping, put a bib on him and monitor the bleed, which may stop on its own. If the bleeding gets heavier or continues for several hours, call your hematologist.

Treating Mouth Bleeds

Amicar, along with factor, should be your first line of defense for mouth bleeds. Ask your hematologist for a prescription, and keep a bottle handy (it's available as a flavored elixir) *before* he starts teething. Amicar is used for mouth bleeds and nosebleeds. If your child has severe hemophilia, use Amicar only after you first infuse factor. Amicar works like this:

When your child injures his tongue, gums, or soft tissues in the mouth, he bleeds. Whether his blood clots by itself or he needs an infusion, blood clots in the mouth have a natural enemy: saliva, alias baby drool. The enzymes in saliva help break down food in the mouth, but they also break down blood clots. This can cause bleeding to reoccur, even if you have infused. Amicar neutralizes these enzymes, allowing a clot to stay in place longer to control bleeding.[3]

Remember, *Amicar does not clot blood*. It prevents enzymes in the mouth from destroying a newly formed blood clot. In people with severe hemophilia, Amicar works only after an infusion.

Most tongue bleeds are superficial—they're just a nuisance. Tongue bleeds can take many days to heal, even after one or two infusions. Why so long? It's hard for clots to stabilize when the muscular and mobile tongue is needed for eating and sucking. Gnawing on teething toys can also dislodge clots. When your child gets a tongue bleed, call your hematologist. An infusion, followed by Amicar for a few days, may be needed. The good news is that most infants have few if any tongue bleeds, and eventually, when your child stops drooling and gnawing, they stop altogether.[4]

LEARNING TO CRAWL AND WALK

Unless he uses a walker, your child will remain fairly immobile until he first tries to crawl or stand, usually after age six months. Bruising may be more apparent now, as your child scuttles on his knees or stands and falls repeatedly. He may catch the edge of a table or crib rail, causing a gum bleed, tongue bite, or bump on his chin or head. Don't be surprised when this happens. Any child can get hurt when trying to stand and walk. Yours will too, but his recovery is complicated by hemophilia.

Head bumps happen when your child learns to walk. Why? Because he has weak muscles and lacks coordination. Plus, his head is large in proportion to his small body. When your child gets a head bump, there's a good chance he'll be fine, especially if he is on prophylaxis. But you should call your hematologist. If your child seems outwardly fine, but he is not on prophylaxis, your hematologist might recommend an infusion as a precaution, or several infusions over a period of several days. React just as you would with any child who has bumped his head: be calm, comfort him, pack your supplies, and drive carefully to the HTC. Everything will be okay![5]

OTHER SOURCES OF BLEEDS

In your child's first year, some bleeds are caused by things you might never suspect, such as blood tests and common childhood illnesses.

It's ironic that having blood drawn for lab tests (see Chapter 3) can cause a bleed, and that your HTC may not warn you. But be prepared! By the end of his first year, your baby will have had blood tests for hemophilia, as well as his routine immunizations. It's hard to locate veins on a baby. Poking and prodding (this sounds worse than it is), holding his arm to stabilize it, or applying pressure with tourniquets might cause a bleed in his elbow or biceps. After your child has a blood test, hold direct pressure on the site for 10 minutes to minimize any bleeding from the site. Then monitor the site for several days for any sign of swelling due to bleeding. Remember: Insist that your pediatrician give subcutaneous inoculations (under the skin) and not in the muscle.

Other unusual bleeds can result from common illnesses in the first year. Many infants get chest colds, whooping cough, or croup. Intense coughing can irritate the throat and lead to bleeding or cause a muscle bleed deep in the abdomen. Severe vomiting can do this, too, but deep abdominal bleeds from vomiting or intense coughing are rare. Pediatricians have excellent remedies for persistent coughs. Check for swelling or discomfort of the throat, neck, or abdomen, or for any sign of blood seepage inside the throat, particularly following tonsillitis, strep throat, flu, chicken pox, or mumps. If you find swelling of the throat, neck, or abdomen, *never assume it is only the sign of a common childhood illness*. It could also be a bleed, either from coughing associated with the illness or from an injury. Well-meaning relatives and friends may try to reassure you by downplaying the symptoms, but it's best to call your hematologist immediately.

5 The First Year

Hemophilia, Fevers, and Pain Relievers

Infants often run high temperatures when they are ill. Remember: Give only **acetaminophen**-based products, such as Tylenol, to reduce fever and pain. *Never give **aspirin** or any products containing aspirin.*[6] Aspirin "thins" the blood by preventing platelets from sticking together, and it inhibits the body's ability to form a clot. When in doubt, check the ingredients of any product, or call your hematologist or pharmacist. The chemical name for aspirin is acetylsalicylic acid (ASA), and it's found in many nonprescription products. Avoid nonsteroidal anti-inflammatory drugs (NSAIDs),[7] which also inhibit platelet adhesion and formation of a platelet plug. If your doctor insists on an anti-inflammatory such as ibuprofen to break a high fever, ask for a consultation with your hematologist first.

JOINT BLEEDS

As your child becomes mobile and toddles around the house, he will start putting stress on those wobbly ankle, knee, and foot joints. All this activity may lead to a bump, twist, or fall. It's not uncommon for joint bleeds to start before age two. Signs of ankle, knee, and toe bleeds include limping and favoring the affected leg. Your child may refuse to walk. He may whimper and be cranky without being able to point to his discomfort. His joint may or may not be swollen and hot to the touch.

Try to diagnose what's happening by comparing the size of one joint to the corresponding joint in the other limb. Recall from our discussion in Chapter 3 that the bleeding joint will be bigger. But in early joint bleeds, you'll see no difference in joint size because the blood is restricted by the **synovium**, a sheath of tough fibrous tissue around the joint. Apply soft, pediatric ice packs to slow the bleeding. All joint bleeds need treatment with factor as soon as possible, so call your hematologist. The sooner your child is treated with factor, the sooner bleeding will stop, recovery can begin, and the risk of permanent joint damage will be reduced.

Parents often feel distressed and guilty when their child develops his first joint bleed. They mistakenly reason that allowing their child to be free and mobile, to experience the joy of walking, has caused him to bleed. Try to remember that your child is developing normally. He's learning to walk, and hemophilia naturally complicates this. You can't stop him from walking, and you can't prevent all bleeds. So let him explore and toddle. That's what he's biologically programmed to do and loves to do!

Many parents say that although being educated about bleeds gives them a sense of control, reading about all the possibilities can frighten them. Yes, it does seem intense and scary. But put your feelings aside for a moment, and focus on your child's health. Being a *responsible* parent means shouldering tasks and coping with your feelings. What's better: Knowing or not knowing? Being prepared or not?

Remember that not every bleed will happen to your child. He may never have mouth bleeds, but he may suffer one or two head bumps. He may finish his first year with no injuries. He may get only mouth bleeds. The possibilities are endless because your child is unique. When bleeds do happen, remember that your child bleeds at the same rate as anyone else; there's usually no immediate urgency or crisis. Take your cues from your child, who may be happily playing while having a bleed or calmly cooing in his crib while his arm is swollen. If he remains calm, then you can too! Even if he cries, your composure will help calm him.

SAFE AND SOUND

After you learn that your child has hemophilia, you may enter the same old rooms with the same old furniture, but suddenly see them as dens of danger. You may think you'll have to remodel your home or even move to a new one to protect your child. "Our street is too busy, the backyard has too much concrete, our stairs are too steep, we need carpeting, we should give away the dog . . ." If you choose to, you'll see danger everywhere. Or you can choose to do what many other parents of children with hemophilia have done—just take routine baby safety precautions and use some common sense.

Protective Gear

These days, personal protective gear is cool and smart. Our children can easily wear protective safety equipment without standing out. But some parents want their children to fit in completely and not wear anything that might label them as different. What are your options?

It's imperative: Every child, with or without hemophilia, should wear a helmet while bicycling, rollerblading, skateboarding, downhill skiing, water skiing, or snowboarding. Someday your child may want to try these activities, and he can! But your child, like all children, should always follow recommended sporting safety rules.

Aside from those safety rules, your child doesn't need to wear protective gear routinely, especially if he is on prophylaxis. Knee and elbow pads are pretty inconspicuous and can be slipped under clothing. Several clothing lines are made especially for children with bleeding disorders; these products have padding fitted into the joints. Some external protective gear, like helmets, will attract attention. This doesn't exactly support our normalcy campaign for hemophilia. Some parents refuse to use helmets because their children will stand out. Others think their toddlers should always wear helmets, to help reduce parents' stress levels and encourage them to focus on fun instead of worrying about injuries. Some parents insist on helmets only at playtime, during the learning-to-walk stage, or on asphalt playgrounds.

Ultimately, your decision about gear and when to wear it will be personal: a function of your family beliefs, your concerns, and your child's activity level. Do what's best for your child so he can explore his environment safely and have fun!

Be Alert!

Despite our emphasis on normalcy and your ever-watchful eye, your child should have identification to let others know he has hemophilia. This is important if your child is injured away from home, or if you are in a car accident or unable to communicate with others in a crisis. Your child should wear some type of medical identification.

Medical IDs, available in the form of a bracelet, anklet, or necklace, will have his medical condition inscribed on the back, often with a phone number for the service company that provides it, such as **MedicAlert**.[8] Any physician or ER staff member can call the company's 24-hour number for your child's specific medical treatment information. While your child is an infant, don't use a necklace. Attach the medical ID bracelet to his ankle, or clip it to his jacket. Place a medical ID sticker on your car window. Consider marking your stroller and car seats with tags providing medical information.

Be alert to other ways you can protect your child. Always strap your child safely in a car seat or booster seat, and always in the back seat, away from air bags. Invest in a good car seat because it could save your child's life. Be sure it's properly installed: 80% of car seats are improperly installed. Your local firefighters or police can professionally install them for free. *No child should ever be allowed to ride unrestrained in a moving car*, even if you're just going around the block. Most car accidents happen within a few miles of home. Car accidents are the leading cause of death in all children under age five, and many states mandate the use of car seats. And don't forget—always use seatbelts yourself.

Modifying the Environment

An alternative to padding your child from head to toe is modifying his environment to make it safer. Of course, it's impossible to create a completely safe environment; accidents and bleeds will happen. But just as babies need cuddling, they need to explore.

Babies explore their environment to find old Cheerios under the counter, tablecloths to pull, or cabinet doors to test. All their learning comes through their senses, so they need to touch, smell, hear, and see everything. The more your child explores, the stronger his curiosity grows, and the more he learns. The worst thing you can do is shut off exploration because you want him to be safe. Instead, encourage exploration, and make your rooms safer.

Invest in carpeting, which can reduce bruises, head bumps, and wear and tear on the knees. If you have hardwood floors, your child should wear sneakers, footed sleepers, or socks with rubber soles for traction. If you use an area or throw rug, make sure it has rubber padding to prevent it from acting like Aladdin's magic carpet!

You may want to get rid of the number-one offender: the coffee table. Some parents who use a coffee table pad its edges and those of the fireplace hearth or large television or media storage stand.

Even if you take no special precautions, always remember that many bleed-causing accidents occur when your child is tired or sick. Fatigue reduces your child's muscle strength and coordination. Buckling knees and stumbling steps can lead to head bumps and mouth cuts. When it's late and he's tired, clear objects out of his path, put pads on him, move the coffee table—or just bundle him off to bed!

THE FIRST INFUSION

All this creeping, crawling, toddling, climbing, and running keeps your baby growing and keeps you exhausted. This means you're doing a good job and raising a normal child. A normal baby with hemophilia may have his first bleed as a result of this activity. If it's a bruise, don't worry. If it's a joint or muscle bleed, he may need his first infusion.

The first infusion is a milestone. It really confirms that your child has hemophilia. It's memorable, too, because of the associated strong emotions: your child is hurt, and you must scurry to the HTC or ER and face the infusion. Infusions aren't normally difficult, but in the first year, they rarely go smoothly. Why? It's hard to find a vein in an infant, even for the most experienced medical staff. Usually this means several needlesticks.

Many mothers say that the first few infusions were more difficult for them than for their babies. It's hard to stay calm and be helpful when your baby screams and you can't relieve his fear or pain, at least until a vein is found and the medicine flows in. Forgetting that babies are pros at screaming, parents may feel guilty for allowing the injury to happen, especially if it seemed preventable.

You have prepared for this day, but actually being there—with your child crying—seems to wipe out all knowledge, rational thinking, and capacity for politeness. You only want the hurting and needlesticks to stop. Things seem better the moment the vein is found and the needle slips in. Everyone sighs with relief (except your child, of course, who swears vengeance by continuing to cry). A sense of control and peace returns. Minutes later, it's over, and you're able to hold and comfort your child.

If your child has a port (see Chapter 7), his infusions during the first few years may differ completely from infusions without a port. Ports offer more control and usually less struggling during infusions. Not every child is a candidate for a port, so talk to your doctor about using a port versus **peripheral** infusions (those done on the outside of the skin into the vein).

> **The First Infusion**
> Eric had his first infusion when he was three months old. We noticed an elongated dark purple mark in the middle of his right bicep. It was frightening, as this was our first reality check in the world of hemophilia. We called our hematologist right away, and he told us to bring Eric into the hospital. I was nervous because I thought that infusions were extremely painful and traumatic.
>
> We arrived at the hospital and waited while the nurse went next door and prepared the room. We were so naïve that we didn't even know what she was doing. She came in with a smile and said, "OK, we're ready for Eric." I wanted to run the other way with my baby! We carried him in and placed him on the table. The nurse put a tourniquet on his little arm, quickly found a vein, pushed the needle in, and the liquid in the syringe went into his arm. She undid the tourniquet and said brightly, "We're all done!"
>
> "That's it?" I asked in amazement. I couldn't believe that everything I had read about infusions was so horrendous. I think if I had read the actual steps involved in an infusion, I would have known better what to expect. —Anonymous

HOPE FOR THE BEST, PREPARE FOR THE UNEXPECTED

There's a lot you can do to prepare for the first infusion, and most of it focuses on emotional concerns. The medical team will focus on the infusion; your job is to focus on the emotional well-being of you and your baby.

- Avoid going to the ER or HTC alone. It's hard to remain calm when you're alone and overwhelmed by strong feelings. You may need someone to support you, while you support your child.
- Your primary job is to comfort your baby. He won't understand why he is having an infusion, but he will understand your love and comfort. Your presence and your ability to stay calm are essential.

- Think of the infusion as a chance for you to be a team player with your medical staff. While they tend to the medical aspects, you can help hold the baby, sing to him, stroke his arm, or even breastfeed him! When you have a vital role to fulfill, you won't be a passive or weepy bystander.
- Put this experience in perspective. Your baby screams and struggles from the overall experience as much as from the needlestick. He's frightened by the hospital surroundings and by the strangers who hold him, and his natural reaction is to scream. It's what babies do best! Eventually your child will not cry when he's infused.
- Babies don't necessarily have to be held down for an infusion. Being held down can be traumatic, and can cause a worse response from him next time. Try keeping your baby seated at first.
- Apply a topical numbing cream to the needlestick site before the infusion. Your child won't feel the needle pinch his skin, though he may still cry, squirm, and fight just because he's being restrained in the HTC. Ask your pediatrician or hematologist for a prescription for **EMLA** or L.M.X.4.[9]
- Advocate for your child if you think a procedure is not being done right or is not best for your child. Request infusion first, x-rays after. Ask for another medical staff person after three unsuccessful needlesticks.
- No one knows yet which vein will be good for your child. The nurses or doctors may need to test different sites. Be patient. Remember to speak up if you see staff going for veins in dangerous locations, such as the wrist or the neck, where infusions might start a bleed or damage nerves.

And when it's over, breathe deeply. Congratulate yourself. You did the best you could under trying circumstances. You conquered the first infusion like a warrior parent—a true milestone!

5 The First Year

SEIZE THE DAY—AND THE FIRST YEAR

Let's be honest: this can be a tough time. You're facing something new, something frustrating, and something you haven't mastered yet. It's hard to watch your infant endure infusions and first bleeds. It's hard to accept that hemophilia is here to stay. This is a good time to reach out to other parents for support, and reach out to your medical staff for advice and reassurance. Remember that doctors are doing their best, and treatments will make your baby well quickly. Life will get better. Down the road, you'll face different challenges and different bleeds, but you'll have more control over hemophilia and you will master hemophilia and its treatment.

So let's put hemophilia in perspective. Your baby's first year is wondrous, unique, and fleeting. You juggle lots of learning, hospital visits, little sleep, and tons of joy. Enjoy your child's first year as much as you can. It's a special time for learning, growing, and loving. Please don't waste this precious time worrying unnecessarily about things that may never happen. One parent recalled sadly that she was so worried and depressed about hemophilia in her child's first year that she didn't enjoy anything. Lack of enjoyment can be self-imposed; so much depends on your focus. The first year goes by quickly, and the good times will outnumber the bad by a wide margin. Have confidence that you will master hemophilia, and know that you will get to sleep again!

The First Year
Chapter 5 Summary

- The first year will probably produce the first signs of hemophilia. You can reduce your anxiety if you prepare.
- Expect to see bruising, but don't worry too much.
- Teething can lead to gum cuts or a tear in the frenulum. Have a bottle of Amicar handy before your child starts to teethe.
- Head bumps may happen as your child learns to walk. Call your hematologist and discuss any that worry you.
- To reduce fever during childhood illnesses, give acetaminophen-based medications, such as Tylenol. Never give medications containing aspirin.
- Treat your child as normally as possible.
- Create a safe environment. Remove or pad the coffee table. Carpet floors. Pad sharp corners of furniture.
- Have your child wear medical identification like a bracelet or anklet.
- Prepare for the first infusion by knowing each step in the process.
- Participate in the infusion by comforting your child. Stay calm.
- Use a topical numbing cream at the infusion site if your child resists the infusion.
- Enjoy every minute of your child's first year—even the sleepless ones!

~ 6 ~

Becoming a Savvy Consumer

We didn't know we had options. We were told the name of one factor brand and assigned one specialty pharmacy. Peyton did not respond to his medication, and after switching physicians, now we are on a new product. It's hard not having all the facts, and with no one giving you options. We found our voice and learned to stand up for our child and our needs.
—Tiffany Holland, North Carolina

After the hemophilia diagnosis, you may think of yourself as the parent of a child with a chronic disorder, a "patient." The word implies waiting, dependency, passivity. Yet you are also a consumer, and that word implies shopping, comparing, bargaining. As a consumer, you are selecting and ordering medicine, purchasing medical services, and seeking the best healthcare value for your insurance dollar. You're shopping for products and services in a multibillion-dollar hemophilia industry. In many ways, you'll act like any consumer: comparing brands, watching prices, and monitoring your budget.

You need two essential things: factor (a product) and a way to obtain it (a service). Your physician will prescribe a brand of factor, and may initially choose the factor brand for you and possibly even select a factor provider to deliver the factor to you.

But ultimately, the responsibility for your child's healthcare belongs to you. This chapter will teach you how to become a savvy consumer. You'll learn how the hemophilia business operates. You'll learn about choices of factor brand and options for factor delivery. And finally, you'll learn how to navigate the marketplace, and how to ask the right questions to get the product and service you need.

HEMOPHILIA, INC.

Hemophilia is multibillion dollar business in the United States. The sale of factor has spawned a large and complicated industry, in which you are the most important player. Who are the other players?

- Manufacturers of factor concentrates
- Factor providers
- HTCs
- **Payers** who reimburse healthcare costs[1]

In a nutshell, here's how the hemophilia business works:

- Pharmaceutical companies develop and manufacture factor.
- These companies sell factor to a licensed pharmacy—a factor provider.
- Your HTC hematologist writes the prescription for your factor.
- You, the consumer, use that prescription to order factor through the factor provider.
- The factor provider delivers the factor to you, or you pick it up directly from the provider's pharmacy or another pharmacy.
- The factor provider invoices your payer the total cost of your factor, and is eventually reimbursed by that payer for each shipment or sale.
- Your payer pays for the product and related medical services.

In this hemophilia marketplace, each player's role can affect price and supply. In a perfectly free market economy, prices are driven by the interaction of supply and demand: high demand for a product tends to drive up price, and low demand tends to reduce price. Consider the high prices of new technologies on the market, like the latest-generation smartphones. Cutting-edge products in high demand create high prices. After a year or so, demand dips—and so does price. Even with limited competition, prices may drop naturally over time, as continued profits more than pay for research, development, and all expenses.

But the hemophilia industry is not a free market. Factor prices are insulated from free market forces that affect regular consumer goods such as televisions, cameras, toys, and computers. Patents, high cost of entry into the market, and orphan drug status[2] all protect the very few sellers and their products from competition. The factor market is an *oligopoly*, with only a few sellers controlling production and supply of a particular product. Hemophilia patients are also a captive consumer market. We have no choice but to use factor from one of the licensed manufacturers.

Even with these limitations, you—the consumer—are the *most important player* in the hemophilia marketplace. Without you, there would be no market. This gives you some purchasing clout. To exercise this clout and to choose the factor brand that's best for you, you'll need to know more about factor.

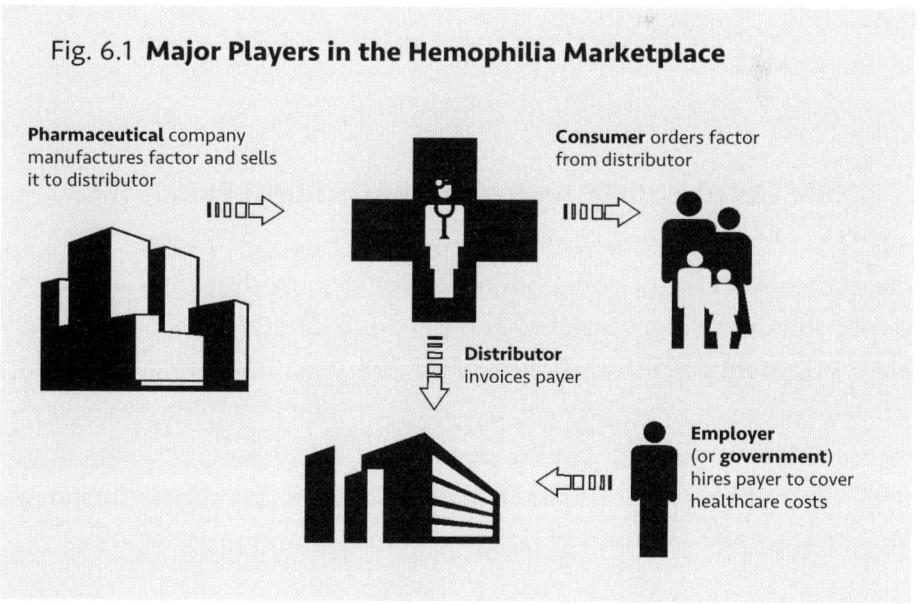

Fig. 6.1 **Major Players in the Hemophilia Marketplace**

Pharmaceutical company manufactures factor and sells it to distributor

Consumer orders factor from distributor

Distributor invoices payer

Employer (or **government**) hires payer to cover healthcare costs

TYPES OF FACTOR CONCENTRATE

There are different kinds of factor concentrates, all with distinct brand names and made by different companies, but all factor concentrates are classified as one of two types:

- Plasma derived
- Recombinant

The major difference between the two types is the origin of the factor, called the *source material*.

Plasma-derived factor originates from human blood plasma.

Recombinant factor originates from genetically engineered mammalian cells containing the human gene for factor (not from human blood).

You might think that recombinant products have an advantage because they don't come from human blood, but some still contain extraneous (unwanted) proteins—human and even animal. To understand the differences among products, you first need to know how various factor products are manufactured.

DIFFERING PURITY AND MANUFACTURING PROCESSES

Plasma-derived factor concentrates are categorized by their degree of purity. Recombinant factor concentrates are categorized by how they are produced. Different—although very similar—manufacturing processes can create products with slight molecular differences in the factor protein and with varying degrees of extraneous proteins in the final product. Here are classifications of factor products, based on varying degrees of purity or differing manufacturing processes:

Plasma derived

- intermediate purity
- high purity
- ultrapure (monoclonal)

Recombinant

- first generation
- second generation
- third generation

Several recombinant factor products also have a prolonged half-life, allowing you to infuse less frequently. The first of these new products was introduced in 2014.

Why are there so many kinds of manufacturing processes? Why not just use one method to produce factor? In some cases, it's partly a legal matter: if manufacturer A creates an effective way to produce factor, then A usually patents the process. No one else can use it. Manufacturer B will need to find another way! So manufacturers have developed a variety of slightly differing processes to produce factor.

It's also a matter of purity and safety. Different products use differing source material and require specific types of manufacturing methods to ensure safety. Due to varying production methods and the type of factor, the relative purity of the final products varies. Purity and safety are two terms you must understand to know which brand of factor to choose, because not all factor concentrates are created equal.

PURITY AND SAFETY

Parents often confuse purity and safety when describing factor concentrates. Purity and safety often go hand-in-hand, but in a medical context they have very specific meanings.

Purity: a measure of the presence of other proteins, sometimes including other clotting factors, in addition to the specific factor supplied in the concentrate

Safety: the removal or inactivation of potentially harmful substances, including blood-borne viruses, from factor concentrate

So purity refers to how much of your factor concentrate contains just factor, with no other proteins. Safety refers to reducing the risk of viral transmission.

Purity is measured by *specific activity*, the ratio of the desired clotting factor protein to the total protein in the concentrate, minus any added **albumin** (a blood plasma protein).[3]

How is factor purified? That is, how are extraneous proteins removed from factor? Factor concentrates are purified by a manufacturing process called **chromatography**. In simple terms, chromatography involves passing a mixture containing factor through a column. The column normally contains small beads coated with a substance that attracts the factor and removes it from the mixture. The column is then flushed out to release the factor, resulting in a final mixture that is thousands of times higher in purity and more concentrated than the original mixture.

Please don't be misled by the term intermediate! These products are still of high purity, although not as high as the ultrapure or monoclonal ones. And note that the various purity levels do not mean there is any less quality control or consistency in manufacturing.

Recombinant products are not produced from human blood plasma. They are produced in large stainless steel tanks, called bioreactors, which contain trillions of cells. Into each of these cells, a gene for human factor has been inserted, or "recombined"—the origin of the name *recombinant*. These genes produce human factor and release it into the culture medium—a nutritious liquid that keeps the animal (or host) cells alive and growing. Although the source material is not blood, some recombinant products contain extraneous human or animal proteins introduced during the production process or added to the final product.

To distinguish between the various production processes, recombinant products are classified according to generation. Generation refers not only to when the products were first developed and commercially available, but also to the presence of animal or human proteins used in the production process or the final product.

First-generation recombinant products, introduced in 1992, use human or animal proteins in the growth medium. These products also contain human albumin added at the final production stage to help stabilize and bulk up the product.

Second-generation recombinant products contain no human albumin added to the final product, but do use human or animal proteins in the growth medium.

Third-generation recombinant products, first available in 2003, contain no human or animal proteins in the growth medium or added to the final product. They have the lowest risk of transmitting viruses.

BRINGING IT ALL TOGETHER: HOW YOUR FACTOR IS MADE

Safety and purity are considered along every step of the factor manufacturing process. For most factor concentrates, the manufacturing process has four basic steps, two of which we just reviewed (sourcing factor and **purification**):

1. Sourcing factor
2. Viral removal and inactivation
3. Purification
4. Final formulation

Sourcing Factor

Plasma-derived products come from human blood plasma. Plasma donors undergo strict screening for disease risk factors, and their plasma is tested for several viral diseases (see Appendix D). Recombinant products are not derived from blood; they originate from genetically engineered mammalian cells containing the human gene for factor. Recombinants are produced in large bioreactors, with human and animal proteins used in the culture medium in first- and second-generation recombinant factor. Third-generation products contain no human or animal proteins in the culture medium or the final product.

Although plasma-derived products potentially risk transmitting blood-borne viruses, all US factor products, whether plasma derived or recombinant, are considered safe by the FDA.[4]

Viral Removal and Inactivation

These methods remove or inactivate most blood-borne viruses including HIV, hepatitis A, hepatitis B, and West Nile virus, making them noninfectious. But no viral inactivation method used on factor concentrate can inactivate *all* viruses. The two most common viral inactivation methods are **heat treatment (pasteurization)** and chemical inactivation. Heat treatment involves exposing the factor to a high temperature for 30 minutes to 72 hours, depending on the method. Chemical inactivation involves mixing the liquid factor in a tank with a **solvent-detergent** (SD) wash for four to six hours.[5] SD viral inactivation is very effective against certain types of viruses, such as HIV and hepatitis B and C, but is ineffective against hepatitis A and some other viruses.

Viruses are also removed by the purification process, especially **immunoaffinity** (monoclonal) purification. Viruses can also be filtered from factor IX through a process called *nanofiltration*.

All plasma-derived products use one or more **viral inactivation** processes, and so do some recombinant products. Yet other recombinant products use no viral inactivation process. Why? The risk of viral contamination is only theoretical, because the product is not exposed to blood plasma.[6]

Purification

This step separates the desired factor from unwanted viruses, proteins, and other foreign substances, to get the purest product containing only the factor you need. For example, when plasma is processed to make factor VIII concentrate, the **serum** may also contain **von Willebrand factor** (VWF), factor I, and other proteins. The higher the listed purity of a product, the fewer the unwanted proteins. Monoclonal products have a higher purity than intermediate products. Recombinant concentrates have the highest purity of all products.

Final Formulation

Even if the viral inactivation and purification processes create a safe and highly pure product, the final formulation—the way a product is packaged and prepared for market—may alter it. In this final step, other components may be *added* into the concentrate! For example, albumin is added into the final formulation in the last manufacturing steps of first-generation recombinant products. Albumin helps to stabilize and bulk up the product.[7] In second-generation recombinant factor, sugar is added in place of albumin at the final formulation step to stabilize the product. In third-generation products, sugar is added to stabilize the final product, and no human blood component or animal

> **Fig. 6.2 Factor Concentrate: Different Manufacturing Methods**
>
> **Plasma derived**
>
> - **intermediate:** contains extraneous human proteins from plasma; albumin added in final formulation
>
> - **monoclonal:** contains trace amounts of extraneous human proteins from plasma; albumin added in final formulation
>
> **Recombinant**
>
> - **first generation:** contains human/animal proteins in culture medium; albumin added in final formulation
>
> - **second generation:** contains human/animal proteins in culture medium; sugar added in final formulation, no albumin added
>
> - **third generation:** no human/animal proteins added at any stage; formulated with sugar, not albumin

proteins are used in the culture medium.

Why anyone would intentionally choose a plasma-derived product instead of recombinant? After all, recombinant factor is the product recommended by MASAC. Why choose an intermediate product and not an ultrapure one? Why inject anything other than the missing factor into your child?

For some people, it's all about cost. Plasma-derived factor, especially intermediate purity, is less expensive than recombinant factor. People who have high out-of-pocket expenses need safe products, but may choose less expensive ones. Sometimes, the decision depends on the type of bleeding disorder being treated. For example, intermediate purity factor VIII products contain factor VIII combined with VWF (the way it's naturally found in the blood) and are useful in treating von Willebrand disease.

WHO MAKES YOUR FACTOR?

As of 2016, 10 pharmaceutical manufacturers are licensed to sell factor in the United States:

- Aptevo Therapeutics Inc.
- Baxalta (Shire in 2017)
- Bayer HealthCare
- Biogen (Bioverativ in 2017)
- CSL Behring
- Grifols
- Kedrion Biopharma
- Novo Nordisk Inc.
- Octapharma
- Pfizer Inc.

Each company manufactures specific kinds of factor products, and each product has a specific brand name. Some companies, such as Bayer and Pfizer, produce only recombinant products. Grifols makes only plasma-derived products. Baxalta and CSL Behring sell both plasma-derived and recombinant products. Biogen offers recombinant prolonged half-life factor. Novo Nordisk manufactures a recombinant VII factor concentrate as well as a recombinant factor VIII. With patents expiring, many of the manufacturers are developing new factor concentrates to expand their product lines and remain competitive in the hemophilia marketplace.

Get to know the manufacturer of your product. Check out the manufacturer's website, listed in Appendix B, and get on its mailing list for news releases. You can also ask your hematologist questions about product choice.

CHOOSING YOUR FACTOR PRODUCT

Time to choose your product! You should know:

- the brand names of all factor products,
- which company produces which product,
- your factor brand name,
- whether your product is plasma derived or recombinant,
- which **assay** (dosing) size you need, and
- why you use your particular product.

That's worth repeating: *Know your factor brand name and why you use that product.*

Who selected your brand—you, your doctor, or both? Could you explain to another parent why you chose that product over the others? Don't leave the decision making to your doctor only, and absolutely not to your payer only. Remember that your payer may prefer to reimburse the least expensive product and not necessarily the best for you. Decide with your physician which product is best for your child. One day you may need to justify your product choice to your payer. It will help if you can learn to speak the language of factor products.

These questions will help guide you to the best product for your child:

- Do I want a plasma-derived or recombinant product?
- Which product does my child's doctor recommend? Why?
- What is the viral inactivation process for the plasma-derived product I am considering?
- What is the purification process for the product I am considering?
- If the product is recombinant, what generation is the product? Does it have a prolonged half-life?

6 Becoming a Savvy Consumer

- Is my child at risk of an **inhibitor**?
- Do I need an intermediate or high purity product?
- Which assay size range does the factor come in? Does this meet my child's needs?
- What type of **reconstitution device** comes with the product?
- What is the price per unit of the product I am considering?
- Is the product covered by my insurance policy?
- How will the price per unit affect my out-of-pocket costs?
- Which manufacturers produce the factor I am considering?
- Does the manufacturer offer a patient assistance program for providing factor if I have a lapse in my insurance?

Table 6.1 Factor Concentrate by Company and Type

Manufacturer	Recombinant FVIII	Recombinant FIX	Recombinant Inhibitor	Plasma Derived FVIII	Plasma Derived FIX	Plasma Derived Inhibitor
Aptevo Therapeutics		✓				
Baxalta	✓	✓		✓	✓	✓
Bayer HealthCare	✓					
Biogen	✓	✓				
CSL Behring	✓	✓		✓	✓	
Grifols				✓	✓	
Kedrion				✓		
Novo Nordisk	✓		✓			
Octapharma	✓					
Pfizer	✓	✓				

US market only. Current as of August 31, 2016. For up-to-date information on available factor products, visit kelleycom.com.

That last point is important: ask your HTC staff about manufacturers' free trial offers for new products. This is a great way to try a new product. Information about effectiveness, purity, safety, and ease of use is continually updated. And new products are always being developed to make life with hemophilia easier.[8]

> **Whether your child uses plasma-derived or recombinant factor, know these facts:**
>
> - All US FDA-approved factor concentrates are considered safe.
> - No plasma-derived US factor concentrate has transmitted **hepatitis C** or HIV since 1986.
> - Recombinant factor products are generally more expensive than plasma-derived products.
> - MASAC recommends recombinant factor concentrate for hemophilia treatment.

CHOOSING YOUR FACTOR PROVIDER

Factor concentrate is a fragile biological drug. Because it can degrade, it must be stored and shipped properly. You can't order factor directly from the manufacturers. You can order factor only through a licensed factor provider. Usually this means a hospital pharmacy, **specialty pharmacy**, HTC, or mail-order pharmacy.

How will you choose a factor provider? Unfortunately, your healthcare payer—insurance company or government program—often chooses for you. But you can exert some consumer clout by negotiating for the service you want. The key is knowing what each factor provider offers, and then deciding what's best for you and your child. Availability, service, convenience, correct assay, and price are all crucial to your decision.

THE HOSPITAL PHARMACY

This is usually not the best option, unless your HTC offers Public Health Service (**PHS**) pricing (see page 107), and most hospitals don't. Most likely, your hospital simply sells factor the way it sells any other drug.[9] Hospital pharmacies have an extremely high cost of service to support the hospital structure, and many are not set up to dispense factor for home use. Some parents report that their hospital charges well over the standard rate per unit for factor.

If you are ever advised to use your hospital pharmacy, call the hospital first and ask the per-unit price. Do this especially if your child is admitted to the hospital and the hospital orders factor from its pharmacy, instead of from your regular factor provider. Compare the hospital per-unit price to prices you might pay if you used a specialty pharmacy.

SPECIALTY PHARMACIES:
DISEASE MANAGEMENT AND HOME CARE

Specialty pharmacies are one of the chief factor providers in the United States. We often call them **home care companies**. But the terms differ. Technically speaking, specialty pharmacies focus on therapies for certain chronic disorders, and may directly provide or subcontract nursing services. Home infusion or home care companies usually focus on providing in-home nursing services. But both can deliver factor directly to you.

Specialty pharmacies and home care services have revolutionized the quality of life with hemophilia since their creation in the late 1970s. Before then, patients were tethered to the hospital to have infusions. Now, if your payer approves the specialty pharmacy, you provide a physician's prescription, make a phone call, order your factor, and receive the order at your home within 24 to 48 hours, along with all necessary **ancillaries** and supplies. Reimbursement specialists handle your insurance paperwork. Life is good!

Specialty pharmacies stock most brands of factor, and usually can provide a size or assay that closely mirrors what you need for your child's infusions (if your factor manufacturer provides the assay sizes you need). Some companies will send a nurse to your home to perform or assist in the infusion process. Over two dozen specialty pharmacies and home care companies service hemophilia, and some are entirely devoted to hemophilia disease management.

Some of these companies donate a percentage of their profits to local and national hemophilia programs and events, supporting fundraisers, college scholarships, hemophilia camps, and educational materials. They develop software to track bleeds, they host workshops, and they help economically challenged families with payments.

With all these great benefits, how do you choose a company? First, find out if your insurance company reimburses for specialty pharmacy services. Then, learn which companies are in-network. Your choices might be limited by the contractual arrangements of your insurance provider, because for the payer, working with a single factor provider is one way to lower costs. And more and more, choice is being restricted; you may face a struggle when choosing a preferred factor provider.

YOUR HTC AS DISTRIBUTOR: PHS PROGRAMS

There are at least 140 HTCs in America as of this writing, and over 100 of them sell factor as licensed distributors. So you also have the option—if your payer permits—to purchase factor from your HTC. How can HTCs afford to get into the aggressive business of buying and selling factor? Why and when would you consider buying from your HTC?

Federally funded HTCs can take advantage of the federal Public Health Service (PHS) Act known as the 340B Drug Pricing Program.[10] The PHS Act allows certain federally funded entities and public hospitals to purchase prescription outpatient drugs (including factor) at steeply discounted prices. So federally funded HTCs can purchase factor from pharmaceutical companies at rock-bottom prices, then sell it to you and make a profit.

In theory, 340B pricing is beneficial. It offers competition to help keep prices down; reduces costs for the government; and generates funds for the HTC to use for staff positions or overhead, which is truly needed.

However, not every eligible HTC uses the 340B program. Buying factor isn't simple. Some HTCs don't have the expertise, space, time, or funding to purchase and inventory all brands and sizes of factor.

Even when an HTC does offer factor through the 340B program, not all the HTC's hemophilia consumers take advantage of this. Why? Sometimes, 340B pricing doesn't guarantee lower prices to the consumer: some HTCs charge the same price per unit as specialty pharmacies, or possibly more, despite their lower acquisition prices. HTCs operating 340B programs typically use revenues from factor sales to help fund their operations and provide factor for indigent patients. And some consumers simply prefer the relationship they have with their specialty pharmacy or home care company reps.

One thing you should know, whether you get factor from your HTC or a specialty pharmacy: by federal mandate, HTCs engaged in 340B pricing *must offer you choice of factor provider*. When an HTC presents its 340B program as an option for buying factor, it must also inform you of your right to choose a specialty pharmacy or home care company as well. Your HTC cannot refuse medical or clinical services because you choose to use a factor provider that is not the HTC.

Checklist for Choosing Your Factor Provider

Ask your HTC, specialty pharmacy, home care company, 340B program, or **PBM** (see next section) these questions before agreeing to use their service or to order factor.

About factor:
- Which brands of factor concentrate do you provide?
- Will I have a choice of products?
- How much product will you provide at one time?
- How are products delivered to me?
- Do you ship during emergencies?
- Do you supply the assay size I need as a single dose?

About pricing:
- How much will I pay per unit of product?
- Do you (the HTC) offer 340B pricing?

About services:
- Are you recognized as an in-network provider by my insurance company?
- What are your hours of operation?
- Are a pharmacist and registered nurse available 24/7?
- Do you (the HTC) offer home care company information?
- Can I use your regular HTC services even if I choose to use a home care company as my factor provider?
- Do you supply ancillaries: needles, syringes, and bandages?
- Do you provide needle disposal containers? How do I dispose of them?
- Do you contract with local home nursing services?
- Is home nursing service included in the cost of product or billed separately?
- Do you provide itemized lists of each shipment?
- Do you provide disease management? Explain what you offer.

PBM PHARMACIES

Another way to buy factor is to use specialty pharmacies through a **pharmacy benefit manager** (PBM). PBMs are companies hired by insurance companies to manage the insurance benefits and prescription drug plans of private-sector entities, such as employers and labor unions. PBMs help determine the formulary—a limited list of preferred drugs that the payer will reimburse. PBMs also negotiate and manage contracts with pharmaceutical companies to purchase the drugs needed by plan beneficiaries like you. The main function of a PBM is to keep prescription drug costs low for the insurance company.

Some PBMs use mail-order pharmacies, which offer cost savings and a convenient alternative to retail pharmacies. Patients usually order prescriptions by fax, email, or the Internet, and often receive a 30- to 90-day supply of medicine through the mail.

PBMs are now powerful players in the hemophilia marketplace. They are multibillion-dollar companies, capable of high-volume drug purchases to receive substantial discounts from pharmaceutical companies. With their vast resources and negotiating skills, PBMs such as Express Scripts and CVS/Caremark now serve most of the hemophilia patients in the country. If you only need factor dropped at your doorstep, pharmacies may offer significant savings.

Some specialty pharmacies contracted by PBMs lack the service and expertise that young families with hemophilia especially need: nursing services, expert consultation on day-to-day care, ancillaries, and reimbursement assistance. Other PBMs have started their own specialty pharmacies to sell factor—and because they have a direct line to the payer, these PBMs are able to switch families from the factor provider of their choice to the PBM's factor provider. Initially hired only to negotiate with pharmaceutical manufacturers to reduce costs for employers, PBMs are beginning to control all aspects of factor delivery. This gives them incredible power over pricing, product availability, and your payer.

ALWAYS ASK THE PRICE

Would you go to a car dealer's showroom and blindly choose a new car without asking the price? Without negotiating a better price? Of course not! As a consumer of an extremely expensive drug, here's a key question you should ask: "What is the price?" Factor concentrate is measured in international units (IU) and priced according to IU. So you'll need to ask, "What is the price per unit?" A lower price might mean lower out-of-pocket costs for you.

Pricing of factor products varies widely. Two patients using the same product through the same specialty pharmacy may pay as much as 30 cents per unit difference! How can that be? Because the patients have different insurance providers, and the factor provider has different contracts. Different brands may have different prices. Plasma-derived factor costs less than recombinant. Prolonged half-life products may cost more than standard recombinant products.

How do you know if you are being fairly charged? *Ask.* Unfortunately, in our gratitude to have this miracle drug that saves our children's lives, we may feel "bad" asking about nickels and dimes per unit. As with funerals and weddings, it just seems crass to question price. But your factor provider is watching those nickels and dimes add up to millions of dollars. *You have a right to know. Always ask.*

Once you know the price of your factor, look at your budget and determine your out-of-pocket costs. Does the product you want or need justify these costs? Work with your HTC social worker to develop a budget that includes the services of your factor provider. Overall, you'll want to look at cost versus benefits, just as you would for any household purchase.

6 Becoming a Savvy Consumer

MAINTAINING CHOICE

Your role as a savvy consumer has never been more crucial. Today, the hemophilia community is confronting massive insurance reforms (see Chapter 15). To maintain the best healthcare, *hemophilia patients must continue to have access to all therapies.*

Factor can't be put on your credit card. It doesn't go on sale or allow 20%-off coupons. You can't exchange it or return it for cash if you make a mistake. Be a smart shopper—the smartest. Everyone wants your business, so use that to your advantage. Always know what factor brand you use, why you use it, how you get it, and what price you pay per unit. Even as payers restrict our treatment options and factor choices, retain any control you can by knowing which questions to ask and asking them.

> **Why We Are So Vigilant About Safety**
>
> The hemophilia community may be the nation's best consumer watchdog group for monitoring the safety of the nation's blood supply. Why? Before 1985, all factor concentrates were plasma derived and not treated to inactivate blood-borne viruses. Hepatitis C has always existed in the nation's blood supply. But when that blood supply became infected with HIV in the late 1970s and early 1980s, the hemophilia community was decimated. We lost thousands of young men with hemophilia to AIDS and to liver damage from HCV. Thousands more still struggle today to stay alive.
>
> Past failures to protect the hemophilia community from blood-borne viruses left our community concerned about long-term safety. Thanks to the efforts of our community's powerful advocates, factor products today are among the safest and most closely scrutinized drugs on the market. Since 1986, no documented case of HCV or HIV transmission has resulted from any ultrapure factor products. Today, NHF's MASAC demands the lowest risk of viral transmission possible, and recommends the use of recombinant factor.

Becoming a Savvy Consumer
Chapter 6 Summary

- You are a consumer—the most important player in a multibillion-dollar hemophilia industry.
- There are two types of factor: plasma derived and recombinant.
- Different production processes create factor of different purity levels: intermediate purity, ultrapure (monoclonal), and first-, second-, and third-generation recombinant.
- In 2014 prolonged half-life products became available on the market.
- Factor brands differ in purity and safety. Purity refers to the presence of extraneous proteins. Safety refers to the measures taken to remove or inactivate potentially harmful viruses.
- Find out which specialty pharmacy supplies your factor: home care company, hospital, 340B program, or PBM.
- Be involved in deciding which brand of factor to use and where to buy it.
- Always know the factor brand you use, why you use it, and the price you pay per unit.

7

Prophylax—and Relax!

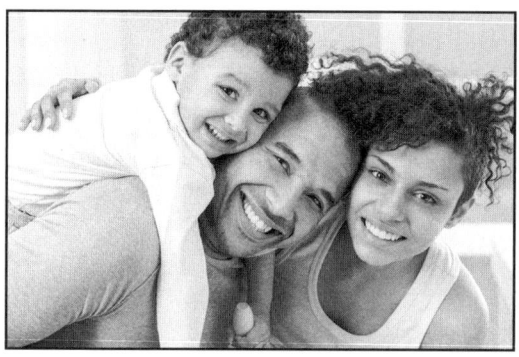

Prophylaxis is like a "sticky pad" under the rug of our life. Now that Cole has factor in his system, we don't feel so on-edge, wondering when the rug will go out from under us. Cole is just as active as he always has been. We have never told him "No" or held him back from normal activity. Prophylaxis has eased our concern about permanent joint damage. —Traci Grant, Washington

Imagine a child with hemophilia who rarely bleeds. That's the goal of prophylaxis, or prophy: to reduce the frequency of bleeds. Prophylaxis means prevention. It's an ongoing scheduled infusion of factor, designed to keep some factor in the bloodstream at all times—greater than 1%—to prevent most spontaneous bleeds, with the long-term goal of reducing joint damage.

Although prophylaxis has many benefits, talk to your hematologist about whether it's right for your child. You'll need to consider these issues:

- The severity of your child's hemophilia
- The cost of factor
- Whether to use a venipuncture or **central venous access device** (port)
- Your readiness to handle this big responsibility

THE CASE FOR PROPHYLAXIS

As you've learned, joint damage from repeated joint bleeds is the most common complication of hemophilia. Repeated bleeding into joints, especially major bleeds, damages cartilage (the smooth protective covering around the ends of bones). By keeping some factor in the blood at all times, prophylaxis significantly reduces the frequency of joint bleeds, helping to maintain healthy cartilage. Over time, your child's joints will be better preserved, so he'll have a greater chance of staying mobile and active throughout his life. NHF's MASAC recommends prophylaxis as the standard of care for children with hemophilia.[1]

Here are the key benefits of prophylaxis:

- Fewer joint bleeds, lowering the risk of developing joint damage
- Lower risk of dangerous bleeds, such as head or GI bleeds
- Less pain, because your child experiences fewer bleeds
- Peace of mind when your child is with friends, on a school trip, or in daycare
- More normal family life (and less parental stress!)
- Participation in a greater variety of physical activities with less risk
- Fewer absences from school or job due to bleeds
- Fewer trips to the hospital for infusions

A huge benefit for families is psychological: life seems more normal. Worries are reduced. Fewer trips are needed to the clinic or ER. Fewer bleeds occur, and the chance of bleeding is reduced. The result? Parents feel more relaxed and less anxious about allowing their children to enjoy activities.

7 Prophylax—and Relax!

THE CASE FOR ON-DEMAND

It's possible to have a near-normal life without prophy, of course. On-demand (or episodic) therapy means infusing at the first symptom of a bleed. Prompt and aggressive treatment of a bleed can minimize joint damage over the long term. But most experts agree that no matter how prompt or aggressive the treatment, if a child with hemophilia bleeds repeatedly into a joint, he will suffer some joint damage eventually. Your decision to choose prophylaxis or on-demand therapy isn't black and white.

You may decide that on-demand therapy is better for your child than prophylaxis for several reasons. A child with moderate or mild hemophilia probably won't need prophy. Another reason is insurance: even when insurance allows prophylaxis, you'll be using a lot of factor weekly. How will this affect your out-of-pocket costs?

Even when insurance covers prophylaxis, some parents still prefer on-demand. Some don't like the idea of infusing factor into their child when they feel he doesn't need it. Others want to avoid excessive wear and tear on veins or don't want to implant a port.[2] On-demand therapy works best when

- you are able to home infuse,
- you are capable of diagnosing a bleed,
- you infuse swiftly and successfully, even if you only suspect there is a bleed, and
- your child has prominent, resilient veins.

If you choose on-demand therapy, *infuse at the first sign of a bleed, even if you just suspect a bleed*. Don't wait until you've determined whether it's a joint, muscle, or tissue bleed. Grab that hemophilia bull by the horns: *Always infuse immediately*.

When considering prophylaxis or on-demand, decide with your HTC team which course is right for you.

All in Vein!

Prominent, resilient veins are often the secret to a successful infusion. Veins can be small, hidden, rubbery, and roll when you try to stick them with a needle. How can you make a vein more prominent for infusing?

- Keep your child warm, or apply dry heat to the infusion area. Blood vessels in hands and arms expand when warm.
- Make sure your child is well hydrated before the infusion.
- Have your child squeeze a small stress ball or rubbery item regularly to build up hand and arm muscles, and just before an infusion to increase blood flow.
- When you find a potential vein, tap it lightly to make it expand.
- Keep your child relaxed, and stay calm yourself. Stress makes blood vessels in the extremities constrict.
- Always access the vein with a tourniquet in place. Learn where and how to properly apply a tourniquet.
- Feel for a resilient vein with your index finger by gently pressing down on the vein and feeling it bounce back to your fingertip.
- Minimize rolling veins (those pesky veins that roll out away as you attempt venipuncture) by using your thumb to stabilize and secure the skin just below the venipuncture site.
- Small butterfly needles, such as 25 gauge, are easier to insert than larger 23-gauge needles, and help preserve the vein.
- Check your needle: not all butterfly needles are created equal. Many people with hemophilia swear by Terumo BCT brand siliconized butterfly needles.
- Apply direct pressure on the needlestick site for 10 minutes after an infusion to help prevent bleeding and scarring.
- Use different veins when possible, to rest your favorite veins.

FOUR TYPES OF PROPHYLAXIS

Depending on when your child needs to start prophylaxis, you'll have four different treatment protocols to consider.

Primary prophylaxis means infusions given routinely before the child has experienced multiple bleeds in a single joint. Physicians disagree about when to start primary prophylaxis. Some recommend waiting until your child has experienced two bleeds into the same joint within a short time, like a few months. Some recommend starting after the first joint bleed and before age two. Others start children on primary prophylaxis even before they have had any bleeds.[3]

Secondary prophylaxis begins *after* a child has had two or more bleeds into a single joint, but before a **target joint** develops. A target joint is one that bleeds repeatedly, generally more than four times in six months or more than 20 in a lifetime.

Tertiary prophylaxis may be started to prevent further joint damage after a child has developed a target joint.

Event-related prophylaxis is recommended before challenging events, such as snowboarding, basketball games, long field trips, dental treatments, surgery, or long airplane flights.

PURPOSE AND PROCEDURE

Prophylaxis requires scheduled infusions. So it's essential to know how much, and how often, factor will be given. Your child's hematologist must decide on a minimum circulating factor level to be maintained—a level high enough to provide protection from damaging joint bleeds. The lowest level that factor drops to between infusions is called the **trough level**, measured as a percentage. The trough level is what's needed to prevent **breakthrough bleeds**, spontaneous bleeds that occur while on prophy.

Trough levels vary from person to person. Some people do fine with 1% trough levels; others may require 5% trough levels or higher. Ideally, your hematologist should do a **recovery study** (also called a **pharmacokinetic** or PK study) to determine how quickly factor is cleared from the blood after an infusion. And you and your hematologist must decide how often prophylactic infusions will be administered: possibly once a day (sometimes for children with inhibitors) to once every two weeks (for children with hemophilia B, using prolonged half-life factor).

If your child has factor IX deficiency, he'll receive prophylactic infusions less often than a child with factor VIII deficiency. This is because factor IX has a longer half-life. Here are two common dosing schedules for prophylaxis using a standard (not prolonged half-life) factor product:

- 25 to 40 factor VIII units per kilogram of body weight three times per week (1 kg = 2.2 lb.)
- 25 to 40 factor IX units per kilogram of body weight two times per week

These dosage schedules don't prevent all bleeds, but they will reduce severity and frequency of breakthrough bleeds. The dosage should be tailored to your child's individual bleeding patterns and how long factor lasts in his bloodstream—something the recovery study will reveal. Children with severe hemophilia who are not on prophy will have spontaneous bleeds. Children on prophy should not have spontaneous bleeds. If they do, their factor dose may need to be increased or infused more often, or they may need to be checked for inhibitors.

Prophylaxis essentially changes your child's bleeding patterns to what a person with moderate or mild hemophilia would experience: that is, he may get a bleed only following an injury. Remember, not all bleeds are eliminated!

Dosage isn't a simple mathematical formula. One treatment **regimen** may not be a cure-all. Your hematologist may need to adjust the factor dosage or the frequency of infusions until you find one that's right for your child, considering his activity level, half-life of factor in his bloodstream, and bleeding pattern.

Prophylactic infusions are most effective when given in the morning. But for convenience—and sometimes because they're unaware—parents may prefer to give a prophylactic infusion the night before it's scheduled. Perhaps their child is calmer at night, or schedules are less hectic. Why is this a problem? Remember: factor degrades, or breaks down, over time. After 8 to 12 hours, only half of the infused standard factor VIII is still active. It's like the value of eating breakfast: eating a lot of food at night won't help you get through the next morning if you skip breakfast.

- Infusing at night means that when your child awakens in the morning, only *half of his infused factor* may still be working.
- Infusing in the morning means that your child will have more factor available when he is most active, providing added safety and reducing the likelihood of a bleed.

WHEN TO START PROPHYLAXIS

Prophylaxis is usually recommended for children with severe hemophilia who have less than 1% factor active in the bloodstream. A child with moderate hemophilia might be considered for prophy if he shows a frequent, consistent bleeding pattern or target joint. But simply having severe hemophilia doesn't mean you're eligible for prophy. As you'll see, many considerations apply.

It seems that children with hemophilia should ideally be started on primary or secondary prophylaxis soon after they become mobile. The goal is to prevent as many bleeds as possible and to preserve developing joints. But it's not so clear-cut. Even experienced hematologists don't often agree on when to start a child on prophy.

WAIT AND SEE

Some physicians recommend waiting to start prophy until a child has an established bleeding pattern. If a child has had two bleeds into the same joint, then he should receive prophylaxis. The logic is that some children may not bleed like textbook cases; some children with severe hemophilia bleed only once a month or even less often. Why pump them full of thousands of units of factor regularly, for years, when they may not need it?

It's possible to raise a child with hemophilia using on-demand therapy and minimize joint damage. How? The parent must treat aggressively and consistently, and make sure the child exercises regularly to maintain strong muscles to protect joints. When parents and hematologist decide to wait and see whether prophylaxis is necessary, parents can spend time being trained to monitor closely for signs of repeated bleeds, bleeding patterns, and target joints. Wait and see works only when parents are responsible and know when to report to the hematologist that the approach needs to change to prophylaxis.

ASAP

Some physicians believe that prophylaxis should begin before the first joint bleed, before or soon after a baby starts walking. The idea is that even one major joint bleed can cause permanent damage. Though some people with severe hemophilia who are not on prophy reach adulthood suffering little joint damage, it's impossible to predict who they will be.

There is agreement in one area: most physicians recommend that as soon as a target joint is identified or even probable, the child should

7 Prophylax—and Relax!

be placed on prophylaxis immediately. This is providing that other criteria are met, such as adequate insurance coverage and well-trained parents. Some physicians recommend that if the child has a strong history of joint bleeds, prophy should be started to prevent what's likely to happen again.

CENTRAL VENOUS ACCESS DEVICES: PRESERVING YOUR CHILD'S VEINS

To start prophylaxis, you need to determine whether your child's veins can handle the increased infusions. Typically, infusions are given through peripheral needlesticks in the hand or elbow. Can you administer factor three times a week when your child's veins are fragile or hard to find, or when he is too young to cooperate?

If the answer is no, then you might consider a **central venous access device** (**CVAD**). CVADs are small, flexible tubes (catheters) threaded into large veins; they allow for infusions without venipuncture. These devices protect your child's tender veins and prevent scarring and scar-tissue buildup. There are two general types of CVADs:

- External devices, also called central lines (brand names include Hickman and Broviac)
- Internal devices, also called ports

External devices

These CVADs are called "external" because tubing from the device protrudes outside the skin. The tubing is taped up and covered with a bandage when not in use. These devices should not get wet, so most often they are covered with a sterile, transparent, semipermeable dressing (like 3M Tegaderm) that allows the child to shower or bathe without getting the dressing wet.

Internal devices

Internal CVADs are called ports. They are completely embedded beneath the skin. Since there are no external parts, internal CVADs require no bandage and allow for normal activities. Because they're so convenient, ports have become the preferred CVAD.

Here's how a port works: A small metal reservoir with a silicone top is implanted in the upper chest (or sometimes under the arm or in the arm) in a port pocket, a surgical space made in the fat or pectoral muscle for placement of the port. Then a catheter (tubing) from the reservoir is surgically implanted in a deep vein in the chest. Implanting the device requires surgery under local or general anesthesia, and usually takes about one hour, followed by a brief hospital stay. Once a port is implanted, it is accessed for infusing factor by putting a needle through disinfected skin into the bump (the port) under the skin. The factor is then pushed into the port with a syringe, running into the reservoir and directly into the vein. The silicone rubber top of the port is self-sealing, and special non-coring Huber needles must be used to avoid damaging the port. Most ports have a lifespan of three to five years.

Ports can make prophylaxis easier and your life less stressful. Ports have advantages over regular needlesticks and external CVADs:

- No searching for veins with each infusion.
- Veins are protected from scarring.
- Your child can go swimming, which isn't possible with external devices.
- The port is less noticeable.
- Prophylactic infusions become less stressful.

The decision to insert a port requires careful planning. Your child will need surgery, a recovery period, and careful monitoring of the port site. You'll need to recognize the symptoms of complications. Your HTC can explain all the details once you make the decision.

7 Prophylax—and Relax!

PORT IMPLANTATION SURGERY

Port implantation might be your child's first surgery, and your hematologist and HTC team will discuss it with you.

The surgery is straightforward and brief, between 45 and 60 minutes. Afterward, your child will be monitored in the hospital, and he'll have infusions to keep his factor levels high while he heals. With the guidance of your HTC staff, you'll be able to monitor your child at home following the surgery to observe signs of infection or bleeding.

COMPLICATIONS: HARD TO PORT

Compared to doing peripheral needlesticks, infusion by port is more complicated. Accessing a port requires special care; and there are risks, including port infections, skin breakdown, and the risk of blood clots.

To prevent introducing bacteria into the port, it's essential to follow strict **aseptic** technique. To the body, a port is foreign material. Unlike the body's own cells, foreign substances make good surfaces where bacteria can colonize. And bacteria that colonize surfaces such as ports often form biofilms—colonies of bacteria that are resistant to the body's **immune system** and to antibiotics. There are two main types of port bacterial infections:

Pocket infection. This happens when the port site itself becomes infected. Symptoms may include fever, redness at the port site, and swelling over and around the port.

Port catheter or reservoir infection. This gives bacteria a direct, continuous path to the bloodstream, and offers the bacteria protection from the immune system and antibiotics. Symptoms may include fever, chills, and low blood pressure. In some cases, symptoms may occur only after an infusion.

These bacterial infections can be serious. Although they are sometimes treatable with antibiotics, they can be fatal if not caught early and properly treated. If the infection doesn't respond to antibiotic treatment, the port must be removed to allow the body and antibiotics to clear the infection and promote healing. Ports that are accessed more often (for example, in people with inhibitors) have a higher risk of port infection (see Chapter 14).

Besides infections, there are other concerns with ports:

- The skin around the port may get irritated from the constant tape and dressing changes.
- Skin erosion (thinning and breakdown of the skin over the site of the port reservoir) can happen when a reservoir is placed too close to the skin surface. And in severe cases, the port may emerge through the skin, becoming partly exposed. This requires removal of the port to allow healing.
- Bleeding can occur within the port pocket.
- **Deep vein thrombosis** (DVT) can happen when a blood clot forms in one of the large veins. These clots can develop when a collection of fibrin protein (a fibrin sheath) forms on the CVAD catheter; this can also activate blood platelets, causing them to stick together (platelet adhesion) and form a clot in the vein. This clot may stay in the vein or migrate to other areas of the body, reducing or blocking blood flow. In some cases, the body can compensate for decreased blood flow in a vein as a result of the blood clot by developing collateral (secondary) veins to reroute the blood flow around the clot. A child's body can develop collateral veins quickly—in just months—and may experience few or no outward signs of DVT. But because the clot can migrate to other areas of the body, DVT is a serious condition that needs immediate medical attention.[4]
- The opening of the catheter may become blocked by a fibrin sheath.

- The catheter may become separated from the reservoir.

If you're considering a port, discuss these issues with your HTC team:

- Ports require surgery to implant and to remove.
- Implantation may cost several thousand dollars.
- About one-third of children with ports develop a port infection, which can lead to serious bacterial infection in the bloodstream.
- About one-third of children with ports develop a deep vein thrombosis (DVT), a blood clot that may close off the port or block blood flow through a deep vein.
- Ports require a time-consuming aseptic technique before and after infusing.
- At what point will your child no longer use a port?

WHEN TO REMOVE THE PORT

How long should a port remain in place? Ports are used mainly to ease venous access and preserve veins. If your child has good veins, he may not need a port. Or he may need a port for only a few years, until his veins have developed enough so that venipunctures can be rotated among different veins, preventing scar-tissue buildup and damage to the vein.[5]

A port may be removed sooner than planned if your child has complications: infection, DVT, skin breakdown, or bleeding at the port site. After healing has taken place, another port might be implanted.[6] Permanent removal of the port is a decision for you and your hematologist, probably based on your child's history of port infections or DVTs and the state of his veins.

THE PRICE OF PERFECTION

Prophylaxis is extremely expensive in the short term. A child on prophy could use more than $1 million in factor by the time he turns 10. You'll need to monitor your out-of-pocket costs to make sure you can afford it.

There's another way to look at prophylaxis and cost. Even though prophy is expensive, consider how much money can be saved later in life. Arguably, without prophy, your child could develop target joints and suffer major joint damage. Or he could have an intracranial hemorrhage. Joint damage may harm his quality of life and may require surgical interventions, perhaps even a joint replacement—all costing a tremendous amount.[7] The money you spend today could be a huge investment because your child's quality of life will be high, now and in the future.

PROPHYLAXIS IS YOUR RESPONSIBILITY TOO

Prophy isn't for everyone. You must meet your HTC's requirements, which include your level of commitment and ability to carefully follow the treatment regimen.

Your child also has to meet some requirements. Your HTC staff will consider the condition of his veins: are they large and prominent? Staff may also consider his emotional tolerance. Imagine transitioning from 35 on-demand infusions per year to 155 infusions per year on prophy. This can disrupt a child's life. Yet infusions become routine and easier over time, and bring a sense of normalcy to hemophilia.

Your responsibilities are crucial:

- You must be educated and trained in properly accessing the port. Your HTC or home healthcare nurse can teach you.

- You must comply with the infusion schedule and follow the treatment regimen carefully. If the regimen doesn't work, or you can't comply for some reason, meet with your HTC team to determine a better schedule.
- You must keep accurate records of all infusions.
- You should have your regimen monitored by your HTC, including regular testing of your child's blood.
- You must know the symptoms of infection and be able to respond quickly.
- You must follow aseptic technique of the port site to prevent infection.

WEANING OFF PROPHYLAXIS

The time may come when your teen or young adult doesn't want to do prophy anymore. How should parents prepare their child when the time comes to wean him?

A young child ending prophy has plenty of time to learn about hemophilia and bleeding as he develops his muscles and explores new activities. But a 20-year-old taken off prophy may need to learn how to read his body, and how to detect bleeds by the tingling sensation (the aura) or other symptoms. You can help him prepare. Have him speak to his HTC staff or to another young adult with hemophilia. Encourage him to treat himself on-demand aggressively. Tell him not to wait until he's sure it's a bleed. When in doubt, infuse.

Even without prophylaxis, compared to children of an earlier era, children with hemophilia today face a bright future. We have great products; knowledgeable physicians, nurses, and social workers; excellent programs for children with hemophilia; and in-depth resources. Take advantage of all your community has to offer, and if that includes prophylaxis, so much the better!

Questions to Ask When Considering Prophylaxis

- What type of prophylaxis should my child use—primary, secondary, tertiary, or event-related?
- Why should we do it?
- What are the benefits? Are there risks?
- How long will my child continue prophylaxis?
- Which product should my child use?
- How will I access the veins? Will I use a port?
- Who will administer the prophylaxis?
- Will I be able to comply with the schedule of infusions?
- Do I know the symptoms of a port infection?
- Do I know what to do when I suspect an infection?
- Do I know the symptoms of DVT?
- Does my insurance cover prophylaxis?
- What are my estimated out-of-pocket costs?

Prophylas–and Relax!
Chapter 7 Summary

- Prophylaxis is the scheduled infusion of clotting factor, designed to keep factor levels high enough in the bloodstream to prevent most, if not all, spontaneous bleeds.
- To effectively treat prophylactically, you must know how much factor to infuse and how often.
- Factor infusions for prophylaxis are most effective when given in the morning.
- There are four kinds of prophylaxis: primary, secondary, tertiary, and event-related.
- Primary prophylaxis means starting regular factor infusions, on a set schedule, before a child has experienced more than two bleeds into a single joint.
- To do prophylaxis, your child may need to have a port implanted.
- Ports require meticulous care, and they carry the risk of blood infection and DVT.
- Prophylaxis is extremely expensive. Make sure your insurance covers it and you can manage your out-of-pocket costs.
- Prophylaxis (and ports) won't last forever for your child. Teach him about hemophilia and how to detect bleeds.

8

Fostering Healthy Self-Esteem

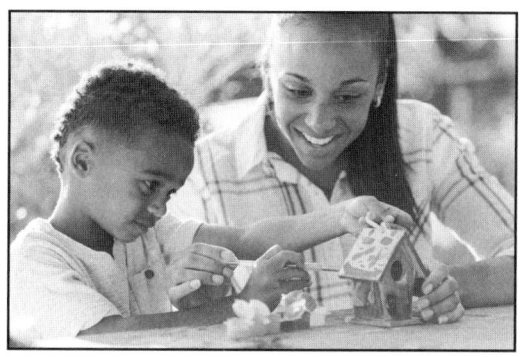

When Justin was one year old, I put mattresses on the floor and padding on corners throughout my house. It was a waste of time. I learned that a child with hemophilia will get hurt; it's impossible to prevent all accidents. Let your child go, and let him learn his limitations. I know this is the hardest thing to do, but it is so important not to overprotect your child, so he can develop normally into an independent adult. —Annette Allen, Arkansas

At age two, your child is just learning self-control. His emerging abilities to speak, run, and do things by himself will one day fulfill his destiny to become independent of you. He swells with pride when adults compliment him on how "big" he is because he can go to the bathroom alone or feed and dress himself. He looks to you, his parent, to notice him, react to him positively, accept his raw emotions, and love him unconditionally. Your child is starting to form self-esteem.

Self-esteem refers to our feelings and thoughts about our personal value and capabilities: in other words, our self-worth. Healthy self-esteem is based on our ability to assess ourselves realistically—skills, strengths, failures, limitations—and to accept ourselves as worthy.

Positive self-esteem means that we value ourselves unconditionally.

The basis for healthy self-esteem forms early. One of its chief components is the amount of control we feel internally, over our thoughts and emotions, and externally, over our environment and choices. People with healthy self-esteem often feel they have the personal power to change their lives, even in the face of challenges.

Yet our children seem to have one big challenge—hemophilia. Facing some limitations and constant medical concerns, they may be characterized as "different" or "disadvantaged" by society and even by their own families. Their self-image and self-esteem may be affected. How can you teach your toddler to care for himself, experience some control over his life, and develop healthy self-esteem? How do you raise your child safely without interfering with his normal desire to be independent of you?

EXPRESSING EMOTIONS

Every child has feelings. Like you, he may feel overwhelmed and powerless because of hemophilia. He wants someone to understand and guide him. Encourage your child to express his feelings openly, and then accept his feelings nonjudgmentally. When you know what he's feeling, you can help him identify his emotions and learn to manage them.

How can you help your child express and manage his emotions? Try these techniques:

- Acknowledge your child's feelings.
- Teach appropriate ways to vent emotions.
- Model appropriate responses to feelings.
- Let your child decide how he feels before you react.

8 Fostering Healthy Self-Esteem

ACKNOWLEDGING YOUR CHILD'S FEELINGS

Acknowledging your child's feelings isn't the same as agreeing with him or approving bad behavior. Your child might be angry or scared about having an infusion, so he may scream. Lecturing him, diverting his attention, or ordering him to stop may work in the short term, but it won't teach him self-control in the long term. Instead, give him some tools. A basic tool to help manage feelings is to identify what he feels. By giving a name to his feeling, you acknowledge it. You're saying, "I understand how you feel."

The best way to identify feelings is to first describe what you see, and then check to see if you're right: "You look angry." "You're crying. Are you sad?" "You're holding your teddy bear tightly. Are you scared?" "That needlestick hurt, didn't it?" Children often lack the names for feelings. You can help by attaching a name to the emotion you see. When you tell him that you recognize what he feels, he'll know his feelings are important to you—and consequently, that he is important to you.

This technique has incredible power to calm your child. When emotions are ignored, trivialized, or harshly judged, negative feelings tend to intensify. Your child may seek more attention. Alternately, it's liberating when someone listens to our negative reactions without judging us. We feel valued: heard, seen, and still loved in spite of it all. Will listening to negative feelings make your child into a little tyrant? No. Identifying and acknowledging feelings gives your child the chance to explore his emotions, with your guidance. Once feelings are expressed and validated, you can work on acceptable ways to manage them.

TEACHING APPROPRIATE WAYS TO VENT

When Michael was young, we used to let him say whatever he wanted during his infusions. No rules—just shout and say whatever you want! Sometimes we were a bit surprised at what he said. But it really helped Michael get rid of some of that anger. —Karen Bishop, Ohio

One way to manage feelings is to teach your child acceptable ways to express them. For example, toddlers rarely verbalize their feelings. Your child may feel anxiety but show it only by breathing rapidly. Or he may act out physically: throwing objects, biting, spitting, kicking, or head banging. What do you do?

Acknowledge his feelings to help calm him.

Ask how you can help, and then provide options. If your child cries at infusion time and you've acknowledged his frustration, give him a choice: "I know you feel angry. Hemophilia hurts sometimes. Listen: You can squeeze my arm tightly when it hurts, or you can punch this pillow. But kicking is not allowed because that might hurt someone." With these brief words, you've acknowledged his feelings, offered him a choice, and set appropriate limits.

Give him a physical way to express his emotions. Punching a pillow, tearing up paper, crying, or drawing a picture about what he feels all give him permission to release his emotions physically.

Teach him to verbalize his feelings. Offer names for his emotions: joy, fear, pride, anger, sadness, hurt, fear, shyness, happiness. Encourage him to use words to express himself. Your child has a right to dislike unpleasant things, regardless of where he experiences them, and even if you don't like hearing about it.

Your child may even express negative feelings toward you. It's painful when a child says he "hates" his parents because they must give him a shot. When this happens, try to remember that he is not really attacking you personally. As difficult as it may seem, try to acknowledge what he feels, not what he says. And acknowledge your own feelings: "I know you don't like having needles, but it hurts my feelings when you say that to me. In our family, you can say, 'I hate having needles' instead of 'I hate the person giving me the needle.'"

MODELING APPROPRIATE RESPONSES

To teach your child better ways to manage emotions, examine the ways you respond to challenges and obstacles in your life: Do you punch walls? Do you remain silent, simmering? Do you ignore problems? Do you complain? Swear? Blame others? Look for solutions? How you respond to life's challenges will influence your child's responses and impact his self-esteem.

Set a good example by modeling acceptable behavior. Begin by giving your own emotions a name: "Boy, waiting for three hours makes me feel frustrated!" "It makes me sad when I see you hurt." Try adding some humor: "When I miss a vein in your hand, I feel so angry at myself that steam blows out my ears like this: Whoosh!" Do something physical to vent your feelings, and then say to your child, "I'm going to tell this nurse how I feel so I don't keep it all inside me," or "I'm going to leave the room and get a drink of water so I can calm down."

Model happy responses too! "I am so proud right now. You sat very still for that shot. Can I give you a big hug?" "I'm glad. You remembered to walk, not run, down the stairs. Nice job!" And model how to encourage expressions of feelings from others and how to show empathy. Without judgment, invite him to tell you how he feels—whether positive or negative—about his accomplishment or disappointment.

FIRST, LET HIM DECIDE HOW HE FEELS

Do you gasp when your child trips a little? Do you jump up and give kisses and hugs as soon as he falls? Do you cry before he cries, or cry harder than he does when he's hurt? One of the hardest things for parents to do is to let their child decide how he feels first, independently of how they feel. They tend to enmesh, or fuse, their emotions with those of their child, especially when he has a medical challenge. Enmeshing means that the boundaries become blurred between where our feelings end and where our child's feelings begin.

Why do parents enmesh their feelings? Sometimes, they consider it their duty to think and feel for their child or to manage his emotions for him. When he tries to express his feelings, especially negative ones, they may rush in to stifle or deny: "Don't say that!" "Don't cry!" Or they may project their own anxiety onto him: "Oh, you poor thing!"

Sometimes parents deny their child's feelings because they're uncomfortable seeing or hearing intense emotions, especially in a child. They particularly dislike seeing their child express anger. Although they may think that squelching their child's expression of anger or frustration will eliminate or control it, they are really denying him the chance to learn how to manage anger by himself. Feelings denied will resurface sooner or later, sometimes as inappropriate or uncontrollable behavior, and sometimes as physical ailments such as depression or ulcers.

When feelings are enmeshed, children begin to lose confidence in their ability to identify and understand their own feelings. They lose some ownership of their emotions. Their feelings are tied to those of their parents, who think that offering instant comfort, sympathy, anger, or happiness will help lessen the child's burden or eliminate negative feelings. In the long run, they may cause emotional dependency, which only weakens self-esteem.

How can you foster emotional independence and greater self-esteem? Let your child express his own feelings about hemophilia and injuries first. Withhold your own reaction for a moment—count to 10 if you must! An added benefit: separating your feelings from his will keep him an honest reporter of his bleeding symptoms, based on what he feels (pain) rather than what you feel (anxiety).

BLAMING AND OVERPROTECTING

One major blow to healthy self-esteem is unjustified guilt, or the feeling that we are responsible for some misfortune. Some guilt is natural and good because it serves as a compass to guide us morally and ethically. Guilt lets us know when we have violated our own moral guidelines. It makes us accept responsibility for our behavior.

But when an unexpected situation happens—an accident, bleed, or illness—and things get intense, parents may blame each other or blame their child. Blaming instills feelings of guilt. Blaming often has less to do with a call to behave responsibly, and more to do with unfairly judging a person's character. Your child should never be blamed for his bleeds. Chronic feelings of guilt will weaken his self-esteem.

Why do parents sometimes blame their children? It's often a reaction to fear. They fear for their child's safety. They fear not being able to protect him. They fear bleeds. Blaming creates a false sense of control: "If you hadn't jumped off that wall, young man, then you wouldn't have gotten a bleed!" There's usually a lot of emotional intensity when parents blame, so the child may focus on his parents' negative emotions and not on his own safety or his own responsibility. He feels guilty for making them angry, the safety lesson isn't learned, and his emotions become enmeshed with theirs. Blaming is not a healthy or effective way to teach.

Fearing for his safety and trying to avoid blaming their child, parents may instead overprotect. When they overprotect, parents try to keep their child with hemophilia from getting any kind of injury, even by interfering with normal human development: "Don't climb on that wall! You could get a bleed!"

How can you effectively teach your child about bleeds and safety without blaming or overprotecting?

Realize that you can't prevent all bleeds, even serious ones. Bleeds happen. You can forbid some activities, but you can't hope to eliminate all risk. Don't blame your child or yourself. Try to emphasize the positive: my child will naturally and normally have bleeds, and I'm being a good parent by letting him be a normal, healthy child.

Realize that you may naturally be overprotective, just as he may naturally need to be rambunctious and active.

Focus on your child's specific behaviors and their consequences, not on his character. Try saying, "When people run with their shoelaces untied, then they trip and get hurt." Take the heat off him by talking about people in general, not about him specifically. Don't worry—he'll still know the lesson is for him.

Avoid saying "I told you so" or even "How did this happen?" This sounds like blame. Focus on the present: the bleed and how to treat it. "This looks like it needs factor." "Should you go inside for some ice?" Eventually, perhaps later that same day, discuss calmly how such a bleed or injury can be prevented in the future.

Teach your child how to navigate safely through his world. Teaching safety rules first, before letting your child explore and play, helps him control consequences through choice. He can choose to accept or ignore the rules, and he'll learn the consequences. He needs repeated lessons—sometimes over months or years—before thinking in terms of cause-and-effect becomes an ingrained response. Be patient! "We have always taught Dustin 'safety first,'" shares one mom. "He can ride his skateboard, but he can't go on a huge half-pipe. He knows his limits but is always testing them."

If you are overprotective, not allowing your child to make decisions and face the consequences of his own actions, you may also be too authoritarian in general. Your child may grow into an indecisive or dependent person, or he may later rebel by becoming a daredevil and ignoring sound medical advice. Examine your general childrearing behaviors and beliefs: How do you treat your children? What tone of voice do you use? Do you smile often? What words do you use?

A well-adjusted child will want to become more independent. And a confident parent will encourage this. It's more important to raise a child with a strong self-image and resilient self-esteem than one with the fewest bleeds or injuries. Healthy self-esteem will carry him farther in life!

AM I DIFFERENT?

When Justin was three, I had no idea that he knew he was different. I thought he was too young to understand. Then one day, Justin saw a movie about boys who had hemophilia. He turned to me and said, "Mom, those boys are like me." —Susan Leonard, Michigan

Around age three, your child will start to question everything. His attention is now focused outward, as he tries to understand how he fits into the world. He may notice that things are different for him sometimes. He may wonder why he gets factor when no one else does.

Will acknowledging that he is different help or hurt your child's self-esteem? It probably depends on how you present it. At this stage, the best explanations have no cause attached: "You were just born that way," or "Nobody really knows why you have it." Preschoolers are egocentric. They are the center of their universe, and sometimes they believe they are responsible for events beyond their control. They tend to view the world in absolute terms like good and bad, healthy and sick. If you try to explain hemophilia by identifying someone or something as the reason he has hemophilia—his mother as a carrier, God, or a special destiny—your child may be greatly confused. When most preschoolers are asked why they have hemophilia, they simply say, "I was just born with it." No one is to blame.

It may be more helpful to focus on *how* instead of *why* at this stage. Ask your child if he'd like to help with the infusion. Creating ways for him to take an active part in his care will help him feel independent and responsible.

PLAY AND SAFETY

Play is more than fun—it's probably the most important way your child learns, and it's a fun way to foster healthy self-esteem. Experience, discovery, exploration, and mastery of his environment all strengthen your child's **cognitive** development. He needs to see what happens when he splashes in a puddle. He needs to know what dirt feels like on his bare feet or sifted through his hands. He needs to know what running as fast as he can feels like, or what's at the top of the slide at the playground. He develops his senses, learns to judge distances, feels differences in the weight of objects, and observes cause and effect. By interacting with his environment, he enhances his coordination and muscle formation, and he acquires new interests. Play enriches his mind and develops his brain.

You may worry at first. Can he swing on swings like other children? Should he ride a tricycle? Can he go down the slide? He can and should! Not only will he improve his coordination and build muscle and bone, but he'll also learn about safety and consequences. And he'll strengthen his intellectual abilities. This kind of learning develops self-esteem.

What if he risks an injury while playing? Your child will learn about limits, and he'll learn to monitor himself through trial and error. He'll learn the consequences of his actions.

Minimize risk and begin to encourage your child's decision-making ability by providing consistent safety rules. From age 13 months to 36 months, your child doesn't make the causal connection between his actions and his injuries. He will not reason, "I shouldn't run so fast because I might fall down." You can help develop this causal connection by setting rules and giving warnings. But be careful how you express warnings: "I want you to stop running now!" can sound like a command or a personal challenge. Don't bring his safety education down to a personal level of *you* versus *him*. Instead, try general rules: "No jumping off the fence." "Going up the slide the wrong way is not allowed here." "All children must hold a grownup's hand to cross the street." Your child is not singled out, you are not the bad guy, and he learns about safety.

Though he still lacks awareness of cause and effect, your child's mastery of running and jumping is improving, and his energy level is rising. This may mean more bleeds! Instead of denying your child the opportunity to learn, play, and explore, try to redirect him to less stressful activities. Always find a creative and appropriate way to let him play, learn, and be a child.

DISCIPLINE

How you discipline your child can directly impact his self-esteem, perhaps more than any other childrearing technique. Discipline doesn't necessarily mean spanking or punishment. Discipline means learning. Indeed, the word comes from the Latin *discipulus*, meaning "student." Nowadays, discipline means learning self-control. Self-control means making choices based on consequences: people choose to obey the law or risk the consequence of fines or jail.

Self-control is closely related to self-esteem. People with healthy self-esteem tend to have strong internal methods of controlling or managing their own behavior. They see themselves as actively influencing their personal destiny. They make their own decisions about their behavior, while understanding and accepting the consequences.

Effective discipline helps children learn self-control by providing meaningful consequences. Consequences can take many forms. They may be positive: bestowing rewards, ignoring unwanted behavior, or giving praise. They may be negative: time out, removing privileges, or corporal punishment (like spanking). When used consistently and appropriately, meaningful consequences shape behavior and help children learn self-control by allowing them to make personal choices.

Many parents who use corporal punishment wonder how hemophilia will change their ability to discipline their children. Specifically, parents wonder whether corporal punishment will cause bleeding. Corporal punishment may include slapping the hand, one spank to the bottom, paddling, or repeated hitting. It's a traditional form of discipline in many societies, including some parts of the United States.

Most child psychologists and child development experts do not recommend corporal punishment as a method of discipline. It's possible to raise a child with hemophilia who understands and respects firm limits, has a strong sense of right and wrong, and possesses good internal self-control without using physical punishment. Corporal punishment can cause bleeds. A parent who causes a bleed could face legal action.

And there are other effective methods of discipline! You can always choose the consequence you will offer.

Ignoring unwanted behavior can be effective for young, nonverbal children. This technique might not stop a tantrum immediately, but over time, your child will learn self-control if no one pays attention to him when he throws himself on the floor and screams. What if the misbehavior, like head banging or hitting, could cause a bleed? Intervene with the least amount of attention. Place a foot under your child's head, but don't look at him. Or restrain him physically, but gently, and don't talk to him. Ignoring succeeds when you forewarn your child—and remind him afterward—that you will ignore this kind of behavior.

Rewards build self-esteem because your child is directly responsible for earning his reward, which might be a desirable object, special trip, or money. The reward must be meaningful to him. He can choose to earn or not earn his reward; this gives him a feeling of control. A reward differs from a bribe. Bribes are under the parent's control, dangled like carrots in front of the child's nose: "I'll buy you some candy at the register if you promise to behave in the store." Rewards are under the child's control: he can earn them. Rewards can be slowly phased out and gradually replaced with praise and recognition within months.

Penalties are negative consequences, which may be physically or emotionally painful. They should be used only as a last resort—if other consequences do not work—and only if you and your child already have a healthy relationship. Penalties will control behavior in the short run, and should be enforced calmly, unemotionally, and privately. Penalties include corporal punishment, time out, logical consequences, and natural consequences.

USING PENALTIES AS DISCIPLINE

Corporal punishment is the least effective penalty because it most directly and negatively affects a child's self-esteem. Spanking and hitting cause physical and emotional pain. Spanking can fill a child with negative feelings: resentment, fear, self-loathing, defensiveness. When children are hit, they learn that hitting others is a way to solve problems, or that a large person hurting a smaller person is acceptable. Spankings may result in short-term compliance but have many long-term negative effects. If you impose corporal punishment, use it only as a last resort, if at all.

Less physically harmful penalties include these options:

Time out: removing a child from the source of trouble. This helps the parent and child calm down, and involves no risk of physical injury. A child can sit in a chair by himself, away from distractions. A general rule is one minute for each year of age, so a two-year-old should be timed out no longer than two minutes. Time out is ineffective when unsupervised, when it lasts too long, or when it's enforced with rage or personal disgust.

Logical consequences: penalties directly linked to the undesirable behavior. For example, the penalty for hitting another child is apologizing to the victim. By contrast, an illogical consequence might be going to your room for an hour after hitting someone. Throwing toys results in toys being removed for the rest of the day. Destroying property means replacing that property.

Natural consequences: the natural outcome of a child's behavior. Natural consequences are allowed by the parents to occur. Leaving toys out in the driveway means that chalk gets ruined in the rain, or a toy truck gets run over by a car. The child quickly learns the consequences of his actions, without his parents' direct involvement.

Too often, disciplining becomes a clash of wills, parent against child. "Because I said so" is often repeated by parents who are tired of fighting with their children, but who really want to win the battle. Like an adult, your child naturally gets defensive when he feels the conflict has become a battle. Try to avoid making each disciplinary action a personal clash. Try not to be emotionally reactive. Citing family rules takes the focus off you and returns it to your child's behavior. You can say, "In our family, we don't call each other names." He eventually realizes that his behavior has resulted in a particular consequence, and he has the power to choose the appropriate behavior next time.

Which discipline method will work best for your family? Choose a philosophy of discipline that reflects your family values, and consistently apply it. Reevaluate if your methods are not providing the desired results, or whenever your child matures and needs new forms of discipline. This should be a family decision, and the discipline method should be suited to each child's age, needs, and temperament.

When choosing a method, instead of looking for short-term solutions such as immediate obedience, think long term. Ask yourself: What kind of child do you want to have in 10 years? What kind of adult would you like him to be? How would you like to see him treat his own children—your grandchildren? Hitting them in a sudden outburst? Screaming at them? Or calmly teaching them to accept the consequences of their behavior? Your child will follow your example. The kind of discipline you choose will have a profound impact on his life and on his children's lives.

Discipline works best when . . .

- Your child knows what's expected of him in different situations. Make rules. "When we go into the store, please don't touch things on the shelves."
- Your child knows the consequences of his behavior ahead of time. "You can play with these toys if you promise to pick them up when you're done. If you don't, we'll have to put them away for a long time."
- Your child is assured that he is loved unconditionally.
- You focus on your child's actions, not on his character. "Hitting your sister is not allowed" works better than "You're a bad boy to hit your sister!"
- You teach, not punish.
- You don't make it a personal conflict.
- You apply consequences consistently, following each unwanted behavior.
- You balance discipline with praise for desired behavior.

SELF-CONTROL DURING INFUSIONS

Self-discipline comes in handy during infusions, and infusions are also prime opportunities for learning self-control. Infusions can involve some discomfort and pain. A young child dislikes being restrained; he may fuss, have a tantrum, scream, or cry. Your initial role will be to comfort your child, but eventually, you'll want to teach him self-control during infusions. Pretty soon, your child will willingly hold out his hand for a needlestick or help with the port infusion.

Before age three, distraction often works. Find an object, story, or video to hold your child's attention or relax him. Starting at age three—or earlier or later, depending on his readiness—you can allow him to participate in his own treatments.

Four methods can ease infusions and offer children control over the process: rituals, direct participation, play therapy, and rewards. All these methods get easier once you've established a level of trust.

Rituals

Rituals are behaviors that are always performed in the same way for the same purpose. They provide stability, and may help your child feel that life is predictable and manageable. Rituals before, during, and after an infusion teach him that things will return to normal and that hemophilia won't always disrupt his life.

Start by offering a favorite security object, such as a stuffed animal, blanket, or pacifier. Deep attachment to these objects is typical of any child under stress and can be encouraged.

Try making humor a ritual. Putting a strip of medical tape on the end of your nose and mumbling absentmindedly, "Now, where did I put that tape?" while preparing for an infusion may send your child into fits of giggles. It's hard to be scared or resentful when you're belly-laughing!

As your child seeks control, he can appear very contrary. He may insist that only his daddy or a certain doctor or nurse does the infusion, then completely change his mind and demand someone else. You'll feel exasperated or hurt, but don't take it personally. Your child is only trying to exert some tiny control over a world largely run by everyone else.

Direct Participation

What's been most helpful with Michael's infusions is letting him have a choice. Would you like to sit at the table like we usually do? Which arm or hand would you like to use for your infusion? Getting the infusion is not a choice, but there are a few choices he can make. It helps him to know he has some control. —Karen Bishop, Ohio

One of the best ways to help the infusion run smoothly is to let your child participate. Even your two-year-old can tell you which hand to try or what type of adhesive bandage to use (Mickey Mouse or SpongeBob?). He can help open the packages of supplies, wipe his skin with alcohol, pat dry with gauze, and count as the factor goes in.

Children aged five and older can do everything in the infusion process, sometimes even the needlestick. Knowing they can do these things, and receiving praise for being careful and responsible, builds self-esteem. Your child will feel less dependent on you and more independent in his own care. Encourage him to participate, but don't force him. Many children are still frightened by blood and the medical procedure. Children with mild or moderate hemophilia may be particularly frightened if they don't receive infusions often and are less familiar with procedures.

Play Therapy

> We made up a story about the "butterfly" and how it comes out of its cocoon (the package), has a long tail (tubing), flies to Patrick's arm, and puts its long silver tongue in him, and how the medicine comes through. Then it flies into its red house (Sharps container). —Mary Haggerty, New York

Toddlers rarely respond to direct questions about hemophilia, particularly about feelings. Try using hand puppets or a favorite stuffed animal when you want to see how your child is feeling but he's tightlipped. With you, he may feel powerless, but with a puppet, he may feel like an adult, a giant. Play therapy gives him a position or feeling of mastery he doesn't think he possesses in real life.

Use your child's natural imagination and desire for control. A toy doctor's kit may be all you need. Your child can practice "infusing" you any time. You can even use real (sterile, unused) syringes, tourniquets, and butterfly needles with the needles removed. Teach hemophilia concepts and explore feelings. Role model, pretending that you're the child and showing that you can sit still.

Toddlers love stories where they are the star, the central character. Stories you create will help your child relax or help you explain procedures. When he knows which procedures to expect, he may not be so anxious. He can learn to better manage his feelings.

Rewards

Rewards are small gifts or awards given to recognize an achievement. When your child shows self-control by sitting calmly through an entire infusion, it's a great time to reward him. Small gifts offer something pleasant to anticipate, and challenge him to strengthen his self-control. The gift might be candy, movie time, or an inexpensive toy wrapped in pretty paper.

Rewards are useful mainly for preschoolers. Use an intermittent schedule to wean your child off rewards. Here's how: Begin by offering rewards after every infusion, every other infusion, then every third infusion, and so on, until eventually you no longer need them. You can say, "Oh, I forgot to wrap a little gift! We'll do it next time." Soon your child will realize he doesn't need to expect a gift in order to sit still.

Above all, to build self-control, you must develop trust. Infusions will go more smoothly if you are honest with your child. Don't tell him he's going to the hospital for just a visit when he's really going for an infusion. Don't tell him the infusion won't hurt. Never use the infusion, factor, doctor, or hospital as threats: "If you do that and get hurt, I'm going to take you to the doctor for factor." Your child's trust in you is the foundation of his growing confidence and self-control. Consistency and honesty are the keys to building trust.

8 Fostering Healthy Self-Esteem

MIRROR, MIRROR

Your child's self-esteem is determined partly by your attitude and responses to life's challenges. To your child, you are a mirror of his self-esteem. When he looks into your eyes, he sees his own worth, because his own identity is still so new. What kind of self do you portray for him? What kind of worth do you reflect? Do you smile when you see him, when he bursts into the room—or do you tell him to take off his muddy shoes? Do you listen attentively when he speaks to you—or do you keep typing away on your laptop or cell phone? Do you "catch" him doing good things—or do you focus on him only when he misbehaves?

You can help your child develop the solid, healthy self-esteem he needs to handle life's joys and disappointments despite hemophilia. Much depends on your attitude and responses, so be a "magic" mirror for him!

Fostering Healthy Self-Esteem
Chapter 8 Summary

- It is your child's destiny to be independent of you. Independence and control over emotions, thoughts, environment, and destiny are key components of healthy self-esteem.
- Acknowledge your child's feelings, teach appropriate ways to vent emotions, model appropriate responses, and let him decide what he's feeling.
- Teach your child about hemophilia by using words and concepts appropriate to his age group.
- Teach safety rules, and then encourage physical activity and play.
- Never blame your child for his bleeds. Guilt and blame can damage self-esteem.
- Overprotection can lead to dependency or rebelliousness. Let your child express his feelings independently of yours.
- Discipline is always a choice. Decide in advance how you want to raise your children, develop a plan, and apply it consistently.
- Use rituals, direct participation, play therapy, or rewards to encourage self-control during infusions.
- Trust encourages self-control. Always be consistent and honest.

～ 9 ～
Hemophilia at Home and on the Road

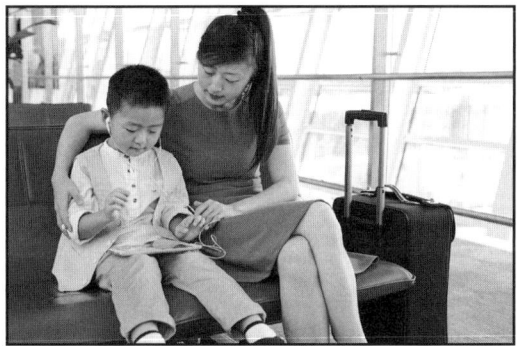

Starting home infusion was heaven! No more lengthy stays in the ER or clinic. Control over our schedules! We finally learned what a normal life was. Freedom to live! —Susan Moore, Ohio

In time, hemophilia becomes such a normal part of everyday life that you think of it as another ordinary household concern: shopping, laundry, haircuts, homework, infusions. But at times, hemophilia will challenge you again. When hemophilia does require your attention, you can feel prepared and capable. These accomplishments will help:

- Knowing your child's individual bleeding pattern
- Expecting certain bleeding milestones
- Learning how to infuse at home
- Leaving home for fun trips

As home life with hemophilia hums along in a regular routine, your child may develop a bleeding routine, too. When you learn to recognize your child's bleeding pattern and unique symptoms, you'll diagnose a bleed faster and more accurately. Knowing which bleeds are likely to happen at certain ages or times helps you detect bleeds promptly. And when you've mastered preparing and infusing factor, you can treat immediately, no matter where you are—even camping in the woods or visiting a theme park. You've become a pro!

GET TO KNOW YOUR CHILD'S HEMOPHILIA

Your child's hemophilia has been classified according to his factor activity level: severe, moderate, or mild.[1] You know by now that children with severe hemophilia typically have spontaneous bleeds (without apparent injury) in addition to bleeds from injuries. Moderately or mildly affected children usually bleed only after injury.

The frequency of these bleeds is only a general guideline because there are individual variations, even among people with the same severity level. Some children with severe hemophilia bleed only monthly, but some children with moderate hemophilia may also bleed monthly with no known trauma. And of course, being on prophylaxis also affects bleeding patterns: some children with severe hemophilia who've been on prophy since birth have never had a bleed! Your child may develop his own bleeding pattern; if he does, this will help you anticipate and prepare for bleeds and treatment.

Which types of bleed will your child experience? This doesn't depend only on his severity level. His activity level, physical makeup, personality, and whether he is on prophylaxis will all affect his bleeding pattern. If he isn't on prophy, you may see great changes in bleeding patterns as your child develops. For example, your toddling one-year-old will develop into a rambunctious two-year-old who is now better coordinated and stronger, runs with fewer falls, and can brace himself fairly well when he does fall. But he's bursting with energy, and his joints are still underdeveloped. This may mean he's more prone to falling than a four-year-old. Your child's unique physical, emotional, and behavioral makeup is the code you must crack to figure out his bleeding pattern, if he has one.

COMMON BLEEDS AND DEVELOPMENTAL MILESTONES

When trying to determine your child's individual bleeding pattern and tendency to bleed, remember to expect some common bleeds as he matures. These include joint bleeds (such as target joints), muscle bleeds, nosebleeds, gum bleeds, gastrointestinal (GI) bleeds, and urinary tract (UT) bleeds. Your child may never get these bleeds, but it helps to be prepared, just in case. If your child is on prophylaxis, these common bleeds may rarely or never happen.

Target Joint Bleeds

Joint and muscle bleeds are the most common bleeds in people with hemophilia. Joint bleeds need the most attention because they can lead to permanent damage. Any joint can bleed, but ankles, knees, and elbows tend to bleed most often. All joint bleeds are serious and require immediate treatment.

Most troubling are joints that bleed repeatedly. No one knows why one child develops a target joint but another child doesn't. Target joints may be related to your child's unique physical makeup.

Target joints early in life can cause serious problems later. Repeated bleeding erodes the protective cartilage covering the bone ends in the joint, eventually causing a crippling form of arthritis called **hemophilic arthropathy**. Fortunately, many physicians recommend prophylaxis at the first sign of a target joint. This can help prevent or slow the progression to arthritis.[2]

Infuse if you notice your child limping, favoring one leg or arm, or feeling pain in a particular joint. Infuse immediately if he says a joint area is tingling or "feels funny"—people with hemophilia often have a strange sensation, called an aura, in the joint when a bleed starts. Remember that children on prophylaxis can still have bleeds; these breakthrough bleeds may require some adjustment of the prophy regimen.

Some joints may bleed more often during rapid joint growth. One parent noted that each time his child had a growth spurt, his joints bled.

Nosebleeds and Gum Bleeds

Most children get a bloody nose sometimes, often from a nose-picking habit. These nosebleeds are usually harmless in children with hemophilia. For children with mild hemophilia, DDAVP[3] alone might stop the bleeding. An infusion might be needed for children with severe hemophilia, followed by doses of Amicar to stabilize a clot.

By age three, your child should be brushing his teeth regularly and seeing the dentist. Tooth brushing and flossing are crucial to hemophilia care. Healthy gums and teeth prevent gum disease that can cause frequent bleeding during brushing or flossing. Consider taking your child to the dentist available at your HTC.

Even without gum disease, tooth brushing occasionally causes some gum bleeding. This usually isn't serious. If gum tissue oozes blood for a while, Amicar may be given after an infusion of factor. Tooth brushing can be reintroduced carefully, with the advice of your doctor, following any mouth or tongue bleed.

Around age six, your child will start to lose his baby teeth. Tooth loss may be uneventful with no bleeding, may produce mild bleeding, or may even require an infusion and Amicar. Body changes are new to your child; perhaps he has never seen blood before. Be sensitive to his fears about external bleeding from the nose or gums. Reassure him that it's okay, and that you have treatments to care for him.

UT Bleeds

You might be surprised when your child has a urinary tract or kidney bleed, even though these are not uncommon. Your child's urine may be tinged orange as the red blood mixes with the yellow urine; it may be the color of strong tea, or may even be red if the bleed is heavy.

Your child may feel some lower back pain. Blood in the urine is called **hematuria**. Hematuria almost always looks more serious than it is. Hematuria can happen at any age, but your child may never experience it, or it may happen once or twice during his development. Kidney bleeds can occur with no visible blood in the urine and may be misdiagnosed as appendicitis. Most kidney bleeds are spontaneous, but they may also be the result of trauma. UT bleeds can be caused by trauma too, but they may also be caused by inflammation resulting from infection.

If your child has hematuria, try not to worry. Remember that a few drops of blood in the urine are enough to turn it red. Stay calm, and speak soothingly your child. Call your hematologist, who may or may not recommend an infusion. Typically, infusions are not given for kidney bleeds because clots in the kidneys and ureters (tubes that connect the kidneys to the bladder) can cause kidney damage or kidney failure. Monitor your child's urine color, and call the clinic every day. If you think the bleeding is getting worse, call immediately. Do not give Amicar during a UT bleed because it can prevent clots in the kidney from dissolving and cause blockage. Make sure your child gets plenty of bed rest, and give him lots of fluids to keep his urinary tract well flushed and reduce the risk of clot formation.

GI Bleeds

Gastrointestinal bleeds include bleeding from the stomach, small intestine, or large intestine. Usually, stools that appear dark and tarry are caused by bleeding from the upper portion of the GI tract. Red, bloody stools are from the lower portion.

Vomited blood may look brown, dark red, or bright red. Brown blood often looks like coffee grounds. The cause of your child's vomited blood may be as simple as having swallowed blood from a mouth bleed or nosebleed, or it may indicate a more serious bleed, such as bleeding in the throat. Always call your hematologist if your child vomits blood that is not from an obvious nosebleed or mouth bleed. And be prepared to go to the ER, because your hematologist will want to determine the bleed's origin. Fortunately, GI bleeds are uncommon in people with hemophilia.

Joint and muscle bleeds will probably happen sometime if your child has severe or moderate hemophilia. The other bleeds mentioned here—nosebleeds, gum bleeds, UT or GI bleeds—may or may not develop as your child matures. They can be scary to read about, but they are rarely life-threatening. Stay cool, and calm your child, who may be frightened at first. Then call your hematologist or hemophilia nurse coordinator, who can offer expert advice on next steps. And remember, all these bleeds won't happen at once! Many will never happen, especially if your child is on prophylaxis. With your experience and skill, and with the excellent treatment available, you'll be able to handle them.

'TIS THE SEASON!

Does your child get excited during the holidays? Have spring fever or cabin fever? Seasons have an effect on people, whether chemical, biological, or psychological. Your child may experience seasonal bleeding patterns: bleeding occurs at certain times of day, week, month, or year. You may find that your child bleeds more often in spring and summer, when he wears lighter clothing with less protection and is more active.

Or he may have seasonal bleeding around holidays. The bustle of welcoming relatives, eating sugar-rich foods, and receiving gifts can all create excitement, and this may mean more activity and increased bleeds.

Accidents happen, and no one is to blame. What's most important is treating promptly and positively so you can get back to the holiday fun!

9 Hemophilia at Home and on the Road

FREE AT LAST! INFUSING AT HOME

The bleeds we've just discussed may seem ominous. But once you learned home infusion, everything changes for the better! Perhaps nothing will improve your life with hemophilia as much as this. The benefits are obvious: fewer ER or clinic visits, less work and school time lost, more time for activities, and lower treatment cost. Infusing your child immediately, in the comfort of his home, lowers the risk of long-term damage by reducing pain and swelling and the need for repeated treatments. Your child heals faster because there is less blood to reabsorb. You regain control of your life.

When should you consider home treatments?

- When you have been trained and approved by your HTC to prepare and reconstitute factor and do venipunctures
- If your child has a port
- If you have home infusion services
- When you feel ready to learn how to administer infusions on your own

Parents have started home infusion with children as young as one year. If your child has a port, you can begin right after you've been trained to use the port. Some families have insurance that allows home health nurses to visit as needed to administer the infusion. Always coordinate first with your HTC. If your child is still young, your HTC may want to see him regularly to be sure he's getting proper treatment and to monitor his development.

Home infusions are challenging in the beginning. How will you know if you're ready to administer the factor yourself?

Learn the infusion process. Your HTC or home health nurse can teach you. Practice the infusion on another adult or on a model rubber arm you can check out from the hospital. Once you feel competent, let your child watch you perform the steps on another adult. Then try it on your child at the HTC, under supervision.

Know relevant medical information. Know the type and brand of factor you use, how to calculate dosage, and how much is needed for various bleeds. Always call your hematologist before administering home infusions for serious injuries.

Be competent and calm enough to actually stick your child. Not wanting to stick your child with an infusion needle is natural, so don't worry if you can't do it right away.

Show good judgment about when to treat and when to seek medical help. An infusion can't cure everything, and sometimes your child still has to go to the ER for x-rays, CT scans, or orthopedic exams. Home infusion is not a substitute for a physician's care.

Understand the risks. Infusing is a medical procedure with potentially serious consequences if not done correctly. You must use aseptic technique to avoid contaminating the infusion materials or site; incorrect handling can cause an infection in your child's blood or his port. In rare cases, your child may have an allergic reaction to a factor infusion. Recognize signs of allergic reaction—hives, itching, coughing, fever, shortness of breath, chest pain, wheezing, swelling, paleness, dizziness, fainting—and know what to do about them. Ask your HTC team for its recommended protocol for allergic reactions.

Accept that you will fail sometimes. Infusions can seem routine—until you miss a vein. You'll be surprised how quickly you and your child become tense when you can't secure a vein. Give yourself a break. We all miss sometimes!

Know how to find (and preserve) veins, or use a port. Infusions are a breeze with prominent veins, but if your child doesn't have prominent veins or if they don't hold up over time, learn how to access more obscure veins or investigate using a port. Try using a smaller needle size, like a 25 gauge.

> **How to Handle Allergic Reactions**
>
> Some people have mild allergic reactions to factor infusions that usually pass in a few minutes. But in rare cases, someone may have a swift, severe whole-body allergic reaction to infused factor that can cause trouble breathing. This potentially life-threatening response is called **anaphylaxis**. When you learn home infusion, your HTC should inform you about allergic reactions and anaphylaxis.
>
> Anaphylaxis usually happens within the first 10 to 20 infusions, or sometimes when a patient switches factor brand. Whenever you switch factor brands, make sure your child is infused at the HTC for the first few infusions so he can be monitored. Although anaphylactic reactions are usually rare, they are common in children with hemophilia B who develop inhibitors. If your child has hemophilia B and inhibitors, ask your physician for a prescription for an EpiPen, which contains epinephrine, a drug that narrows blood vessels and opens airways. This will help counter some of the effects of the anaphylactic reaction.
>
> If your child experiences anaphylaxis, call 911. Never attempt to drive yourself to the hospital. While waiting for medical help, use your EpiPen if you have one.

Some HTCs postpone teaching home infusion to parents who are eager to learn. If this happens to you, ask why. Some HTCs are reluctant to turn over responsibility to the parent. Others fear a lawsuit if something goes wrong. Some simply want to bill the patient for services. Still others assess correctly that the parents aren't ready for home infusions—because of an unstable home environment, a demonstrated lack of responsibility, or a poor attitude. Home infusions are a big step and a huge responsibility.

If you are trained by your HTC and begin home infusion, it's an achievement. But the one person who may not appreciate your new achievement is your child! Children like routines, even ones that aren't ideal. Your child may rebel at any change in routine. Or he might be angry that he can't go to the hospital, where he was lavished with attention. Expect a temporary change in your child's behavior when you begin home infusion. If you're upset or nervous about doing the infusion, your child may sense it. But give yourself permission to make mistakes. Remember that you are new at this, and it takes time to develop skill finding a vein. Focus on your active participation in making his life with hemophilia feel more normal.

RECORDING BLEEDS AND INFUSIONS

Keeping accurate, up-to-date records of each injury and infusion is one of your prime responsibilities as a parent. There are many benefits:

- You'll learn which types of injuries and bleeds are most common for your child.
- You'll learn how often and under what circumstances his bleeds occur.
- You'll have a record of the type of factor he received and the lot number, in the event of a product **recall** or **withdrawal**.
- You can easily share this information with your HTC online.
- You may need records for insurance purposes. Hospitals sometimes bill incorrectly. In this era of healthcare cost cutting, records are your proof that a treatment was needed, and that factor was not squandered or misplaced.[4]

Your HTC or home care company may supply infusion charts, computer software, an electronic device, or apps for your tablet or smart phone, or you can invent your own. Buy a notebook, create a spreadsheet on your computer, or use a software program provided by your home care company or factor manufacturer.[5] Some manufacturers provide hand-held devices that scan and automatically record all information about the product. Log any follow-up treatments, and include any hospital visits and extra exams. Were x-rays taken? CT scan? How many doctors examined him?

If you infuse at the hospital or clinic, tear off the top of the factor box to take home. Copy the information from the boxtop into your log. Your clinic will also record this information.

Someday you'll be giving infusions at home—it's true! Infusions will become routine, like any household chore. And someday your child will hold out his hand calmly while you infuse him, or sit quietly if he has a port. Someday he'll infuse himself. Learn to home infuse as soon as you feel ready and are trained. Nothing will make you feel more independent!

Fig. 9.1 Sample Factor Log

Patient Name: *Joey*   Age: *9*   Weight: *63 lb.*

Date	Injury Site	Product	Units	Lot Number	Comments
6/29/16	Left thigh muscle	"Factorate"	1,000	X0T 456 01	Felt better after 1 hour
7/15/16	Right elbow	"Factorate"	1,000	X0T 456 01	Called HTC, applied ice, rest

ON THE ROAD AGAIN!

When home infusions make you feel comfortable enough to take vacations again, you'll know your normal life has returned. Even if you don't infuse your child yet, you can still travel, as long as you're prepared.

Map Out the HTCs

First, locate the HTC nearest to your travel destination. If you're taking a long trip by bus, train, or car, map out the HTCs along your route.[6] Next, inform the HTC nurse coordinator when you will be in that area. Do this before your trip! Learn about each HTC facility: clinic hours, pager numbers, ER phone number. Find out if your child's name can be registered in the ER logbook, if one is maintained. Provide your home care company with your vacation information—hotel name and address, campsite, phone numbers—in case you need factor and supplies shipped.[7] Have your hematologist write a travel letter to bring with you to expedite treatment at ERs not familiar with hemophilia.

Supplies

Bring your own supply of factor and ancillaries. It's risky to rely on the local HTC to have the product you need; and many small hospitals carry no factor on hand, because of its high cost.[8] If you're relying on your home care company to ship your factor, always bring enough for a few days in case of delivery problems. Bring your child's immunization booklet to prove that his shots are up-to-date if you need to visit the ER.

Luggage

If you're traveling by plane or train, keep a few doses of factor in your carry-on luggage, and, depending on how much you're bringing, the rest in your checked luggage. It's always possible for your checked luggage to be delayed, so it's best to keep as much in the carry-on as possible. If your child needs an infusion immediately—say, at 30,000 feet—you'll be ready. Since 9/11, airlines have restricted what you can carry onboard national and international flights. Call your airline in advance: Which liquids, injectables, and ancillaries can you bring in your carry-on? How much you are permitted to carry?

Travel Letter

Along with your supplies, pack a travel letter from your hematologist. This letter should contain the following:

- Your child's hemophilia diagnosis
- Recommended treatment
- Dosage for various bleeds
- Statement that you are competent to administer the prescription product or oversee administration
- Purpose of medical ancillaries
- Statement that it's safe for your child to fly
- Description of factor as a white powder

If you're traveling to a country where English is not widely spoken, have your letter translated into the local language before you leave. Bring an up-to-date prescription as legal proof that you have a right to carry prescription products. To customs officials, factor concentrates may look like illegal narcotics. This is why your travel letter should state that factor is a sterile white powder and that the vials should not be opened.

Store and Dispose of Factor Safely

Most factor can be stored at room temperature. But vacation spots may be in warm, tropical climates or near snowy ski slopes. Factor should never be frozen, and should not be left in cars in warm weather. Even when the outside temperature is cool, car interiors can be substantially hotter, by as much as 30 degrees F. Remove your factor from the car in winter and summer, and store it in a refrigerator or cooler.

After reconstituting factor, use all of it as soon as possible. Reconstituted factor should not be stored for later use, because the factor might have been contaminated with bacteria during the reconstitution process. Factor manufacturers usually recommend that all reconstituted factor be infused within three to four hours, and any factor not infused should be discarded. Check your product insert for more information about storing your brand of factor. Ask about travel packs supplied by some home care companies and manufacturers.

Don't forget about responsible waste disposal. Never drop used needles in the trash. When discarded improperly, needles can easily pierce someone. Needles contaminated with blood may cause infection. Ask your home care company or HTC for small, portable **Sharps** containers to prevent accidents. If you have no container and you're desperate, use a tin can or locate the nearest hospital or fire department and ask to discard your materials there.

> **Perfect Travel Planning**
>
> - Locate an HTC at your travel destination or en route, and contact it before you go. NHF's website will direct you to the CDC's website for a US list; the World Federation of Hemophilia (WFH) website lists international HTCs.
> - Tell your home care company where you'll be.
> - Check with airlines about which liquids and injectables are permitted.
> - Pack some factor in your checked luggage and some in your carry-on.
> - Pack your child's prescription and a travel letter from your hematologist with your supplies.
> - Pack and store your factor appropriately. Factor should never be frozen or left in cars in warm weather.
> - Bring a Sharps container, and properly dispose of used needles and medical items. Do not put a Sharps container in your checked baggage.
> - Bring your factor logbook or electronic device to record all bleeds and factor usage.
> - Check your insurance for out-of-state, out-of-country, and emergency coverage.
> - Wear seatbelts, use car seats, and have your child wear a medical ID bracelet or necklace.

Insurance

Check your medical insurance before taking a trip. Does your policy cover you out of state? Out of the country? When, if ever, would your policy not cover you? Do you need your primary care physician's referral to take your child to a doctor while visiting another city? If you're out of the country, does your insurance cover medical evacuation? You may want the answers to these questions in writing before you leave. In some cases, you may need to buy additional insurance.

Bring your insurance card and forms with you on the road. If your child needs emergency treatment, you may need to notify your insurance company within 48 hours to make sure that you fill out the proper forms.

Now, Go Away!

Did you think the day would ever come? You know your child better now. You have a sense of when and how he bleeds. You've mastered home infusions, and you know to expect certain types of bleeds. Home has become your base camp, and you're ready to venture out to conquer mountains of excitement as a family: road trips, day trips, carnivals, theme parks, science museums, the beach.

Pack your factor, locate some HTCs, gas up the car, grab your cell phone and some road games, and head into the sunset. Under your dedicated management, hemophilia has finally become a normal part of your life. You've done a great job. You deserve a vacation!

Hemophilia at Home
Chapter 9 Summary

- Learn how your child feels and behaves when he has bleeds so you can accurately and rapidly diagnose them.
- Bleeding patterns may depend on severity level, activity level, physical makeup, or personality, and may even occur during specific seasons or holidays.
- Target joints occur when one joint bleeds repeatedly. Treat joint bleeds immediately.
- Expect some bleeds as your child matures: joint bleeds, muscle bleeds, nosebleeds, GI and UT bleeds.
- To infuse at home, you must know your factor and dosage information, use good judgment in diagnosing a bleed, know how to mix the factor, and have good venous access.
- Record each infusion: date, injury, number of units, type of factor, expiration date, and lot number.
- When traveling, contact the HTC nearest your destination before you go. Bring factor and ancillaries. Take proper care of your factor. Check your medical insurance before taking a trip, especially overseas.
- Check with airlines ahead of time to find out which liquids and injectables are permitted in your carry-on luggage.

10

School Days

The first-grade teacher did a wonderful presentation on how children are unique. With parental permission, she introduced three children in her class—one with severe diabetes, one with cerebral palsy, and Michael with hemophilia. Each child got up and spoke, and the teacher gave information about each medical situation. From then on, the children in that class just thought that the diabetes, hemophilia, and cerebral palsy were entirely normal. —Mary Fitzpatrick, New Hampshire

From ages six to twelve, your child develops from childhood to the brink of adolescence. This is a time of expansive physical and emotional growth and tremendous learning. Your child has a firm foothold on the path to independence. You want him to become independent, and you're proud and happy to see him blossom. Yet you may have mixed feelings as you watch your child enter school for the first time.

Just as life settles down, and you feel competent and comfortable with hemophilia, the rest of the world will now meet your child with hemophilia. The child you loved, nurtured, and protected is now among other children and teachers who know little about his condition, in an environment beyond your supervision. It's normal to feel anxious!

Your child may be anxious, too. School is his first venture into the "real" world. He will make independent decisions about his behavior, and he'll take on more responsibility. He will interact with other children and make friends. With solid self-esteem, knowledge about hemophilia, and your unconditional love, your child will shine during these formative years!

FROM PRESCHOOL TO FIRST GRADE

It's rare these days to find a child who spent his first five years at home full time, and this includes children with hemophilia. If your child has attended daycare or preschool, you may feel confident handling primary school issues related to hemophilia.

Regardless of how your child spent his preschool years, attending kindergarten means that he will be mainstreamed in a classroom. He'll be supervised with up to 25 or more youngsters. Never before has your child been so free to test his limits. You may worry constantly whether anyone will notice that he bumped his head or hurt his knee. You'll wonder if your child is responsible enough to report that he has a bleed.

By the time he reaches first grade, your child may be graded or compared to others. He will begin to learn about his world through his class curriculum, and he'll be expected to keep up with his peers. He may start having homework. If he misses school or homework assignments because of hemophilia—an elbow or wrist bleed, for example—he may feel anxious. Fortunately, given current medical care and prophylaxis, bleeds should rarely result in school absences.

Making sure your child is happy, confident, and healthy is a team effort now involving you, your child, and school personnel. What should you tell the school personnel? How can you promote the best understanding of this rare disorder? How will you explain hemophilia to your child's classmates?

TELLING SCHOOL PERSONNEL

Put yourself in a teacher's place: you have a classroom full of small children, all with differing backgrounds, personalities, energy levels, abilities, and challenges. Your job is to instruct them, manage them, account for individual differences, foster cooperation, evaluate their development, and have fun—for six hours every day! As the school year begins, you learn that one of your students is a wonderful child with a rare bleeding disorder. What now?

For the uninitiated, hemophilia may conjure images of profuse bleeding, emergencies, and chaos. School personnel wonder: Can he use scissors? Can he play at recess? Is he as intelligent as the others? How can I watch him and the other children, too? What happens when he gets hurt? Will he bleed excessively?

Remember how much better you felt as a parent, when you armed yourself with knowledge? Your child's teachers will, too. But how do you begin?

- Contact your HTC. The staff will advise you or even come to school.
- Order the resources in Appendix A to leave with school personnel.
- Arrange a first meeting with school personnel before school starts.

The first meeting should include

- your child's head teacher
- assistant teachers
- teacher's aides
- principal
- administrative assistant
- physical education teacher
- school nurse

Ask your HTC nurse or home health nurse to attend. This lends credibility and a professional perspective. Your HTC representative may also want to meet with school personnel privately to answer any questions they're reluctant to ask in front of you. Your child doesn't need to be at this first meeting, although he should be told about it. Ask your child if he'd like to attend. He can practice taking personal responsibility for his disorder by speaking directly to school personnel about his abilities and any limitations.

Give school personnel some materials to read, but don't overload them with information.[1] Audiences usually recall only three main points of any meeting, so choose which three you want to emphasize. Your first meeting's agenda should be simple and focused on handling hemophilia in school:

- Explain hemophilia, and dispel myths.
- Describe the symptoms of a bleed: swelling, limping, favoring a limb.
- Describe the types of bleeds your child is likely to have.
- Explain the different severity levels, and share your child's level.
- Describe your child's specific limitations and abilities: he can play at recess; he can't be hit in the chest with a kickball.
- Emphasize that your child should be treated normally.
- Supply your contact phone numbers.
- Reassure everyone that they will not have to learn how to infuse.
- Ask if factor can be stored in the nurse's office.
- Provide emergency numbers and instructions in case you can't be reached: HTC, hematologist, local pediatrician.

Reassure school personnel that they can treat your son normally, and they can believe him when he says he needs treatment. They should never single him out, announce that he has hemophilia, or make an issue of his medical ID bracelet or his bruises. They should take normal precautions and observe normal safety practices. Remind them to follow standard first aid procedures for most injuries. This treatment should not be delayed while they attempt to notify you.[2]

Later in the school year, you can meet again. School personnel will have more questions and may be more comfortable and eager to learn, as you once were.

10 School Days

THE TEACHER-PARENT-CHILD PARTNERSHIP

It's normal for anyone to be apprehensive at the thought of a child with hemophilia in the classroom, but it can especially worry the teacher, who bears responsibility for the students. Even if the teacher has some knowledge or experience, no two children with hemophilia are alike. Chances are, yours will be the first child with hemophilia that his teacher has met.

Many teachers have taught children with special needs, and they may be completely comfortable with your child. But for others, your first meeting only temporarily relieves anxieties. A teacher could develop new concerns when left alone with your child for the day. Afraid of injuries, fearing the sight of blood, and anxious about being held responsible, a worried teacher might exhibit such negative behaviors as overprotection, singling out, denial, and overreaction.

Overprotection

Fearing injuries, a teacher may exclude your child from some activities. To prevent overprotection, ask the teacher to watch for symptoms of a bleed or call you when your child tries a new activity—this shifts the responsibility off the teacher a bit. Provide a list of activities that are safe for your child: using scissors, playing on the concrete or asphalt surface, using playground equipment, jumping rope, playing kickball and tag. If you want to forbid a specific activity—like hanging by his arms from the jungle gym after a forearm or shoulder bleed—write a note to his classroom and physical education teachers. Ask them to find creative ways to include your child in an activity, despite a bleed that sidelines him. He could be the assistant "coach" or scorekeeper, for example.

Singling Out

Your child's teacher may unwittingly single him out by announcing to the class that he has a blood disorder. The teacher may constantly remind other children not to hit your child. The phrase "Now, everyone except . . ." directs attention to your child. This is the worst thing a teacher can do! Most children dislike uninvited attention. Too much attention, especially when it sets a child apart from classmates, can breed resentment. Your child could be ostracized or teased by classmates.

If your child must avoid a particular activity (with your approval), teachers should arrange a face-saving and tactful way to exclude him—one that doesn't attack or shame him, or draw attention to his disorder.

Denial

On most days, your child can participate in all activities and show no signs of bleeding. On other days, your child must be excused from certain activities when he is recovering from an injury or bleed. Outwardly, he appears fine, and his teacher may not recognize the need for rest. It's even harder for the physical education teacher, who often hears a long list of illnesses and complaints from children who simply don't want to run laps or climb ropes. Remember to stress that all teachers should trust your child's assessment of a bleed or his recovery, with or without notes from home.[3]

Overreaction

Some people react emotionally to bleeds and injuries. Most teachers model emotionally mature behavior in the classroom, but some may gush "ooh" and "aah" over a child's bruises and swellings, or exclaim, "Poor boy!" This puts a spotlight on your child and can lower his self-esteem. He feels different from his classmates, and along with them, he may develop negative feelings about hemophilia. Injuries and bleeds should be handled calmly and competently, with concern but with minimal fuss.

Teachers are our early warning systems. They provide information about our children's development. Teachers tell us how our children are adjusting to school. They can alert us to signs of depression, such as withdrawal or slipping grades, which may indicate poor self-image or adjustment. They can tell us whether our children are interacting well with others or being bullied. They notice if our children are afraid to take risks.

Communication, trust, and respect between parent and teacher are key building blocks of a positive student-teacher relationship. Keep communication channels open by scheduling periodic meetings to answer school personnel questions. Consider becoming involved in school activities like parent–teacher groups. Volunteer at your child's school. Attend open house events or chaperone a field trip, and model how you handle your child and his hemophilia. Keep his teacher up-to-date with events at home, such as a traumatic bleed while on vacation, the impending birth of a sibling, or anything that might cause stress and lead to a bleed or might be reflected in school participation and attitude. Get involved with your child's school experience to demonstrate your positive attitude and serve as a role model.

SCHOOL NURSE

The school nurse is often your first line of defense when seeking proper medical treatment. You might be able to infuse your child in the nurse's office or involve the nurse in the infusion.

When you meet with the school nurse, either alone or with your child's team of teachers, you may want to find out what he or she knows about hemophilia, and then supply any missing information. Some nurses are familiar with hemophilia, but because hemophilia is so rare, most are not. Some nurses claim to know "everything" about hemophilia so they don't look ignorant!

If you're unsure of the school nurse's understanding of hemophilia, ask your HTC nurse to intervene and act as a resource. Is the school nurse willing to be involved with hemophilia and assume some responsibility for your child? If so, then this nurse will be a valuable asset.

MISSING SCHOOL

In these days of prophylaxis and prompt treatment, school absences are declining for children with hemophilia. Still, you may face a time when your child needs to be off his feet to recover. Don't let your child fall behind because of hemophilia; his education is crucial. Put a plan in place to ensure that he'll stay abreast of his peers and complete the required work.

If your child must miss some school time, alert the classroom teacher. You may want to put this in writing and estimate the amount of time: one day, one week, two weeks? Alert your child's other teachers or aides: special education teacher, art instructor, physical education teacher.

Ask your child's classmates to bring his work home. Many schools are online, and homework can be emailed. Give the teacher weekly updates while your child is absent, and ask for weekly updates on the returned work. Ask for classroom news about special events or new students.

Mark your calendar with events scheduled for your child's class. Can you imagine not knowing that you missed the big field trip to the science museum or the school talent show? Although your child must remain off his feet, he'll want to know about these programs or perhaps attend one after school.

All public schools in the United States are required by federal law to provide services for children with special needs. Your child may have a special need if he finds it too difficult to keep up with schoolwork because of his absences relating to bleeds. Ask your school's special education department about state laws regarding home schooling and tutoring. Ask about a 504 Accommodation Plan. Section 504 is a federal civil rights law under the Rehabilitation Act of 1973.[4]

Depending on the need, a school district may be required to provide these services: specialized instruction, modifications to the curriculum, accommodations in nonacademic and extracurricular activities, adaptive equipment or assistive technology devices, an aide, assistance with health-related needs, school transportation, or other related services and accommodations. Your child might need special environmental changes, such as extra time to make it to class after the bell, or help boarding the school bus. Even if it's only temporary, your child may have a special need, and the law requires your school to help you.

I'M DIFFERENT

The influence of peers becomes very strong during the school years. Your child may idolize a particular friend or want to belong to the "in" crowd on the playground. As peer influence rises, your influence may decline slightly. Make the most of your first five years with your child: prepare him to interact appropriately with others, and teach him how to fit into his new social sphere at school.

When he's with his peers, your child may suddenly realize, "I'm different." He may have been almost oblivious to hemophilia before entering school. Although he needed treatments periodically and sometimes had restrictions, this probably didn't bother him much because he was still egocentric, seeing things from only his point of view.

But now he's one member of a big social group. Although he's still egocentric, he begins to compare himself to others. He wants to fit in and be liked. His new friends may bombard him with questions: "Where did you go? Why didn't you come to school for three days? Are you sick? How did you get that bruise? Why are you wearing that bracelet?" The spotlight is on him.

Being in the spotlight because he's different is probably a revelation, whether positive or negative. He may feel proud to be different—not squeamish about needles, unlike his friends. Yet the realization may be disturbing if he isn't well prepared for other people's reactions, has a poor self-image, or was taught to hide his hemophilia. If he's uncomfortable with hemophilia, he may start ignoring his bleeds to prove that he's not different.

Or he may focus too much on bleeds. It's normal for a child with hemophilia to use bleeds as a way to express his feelings.

For example, it's perfectly normal for a child with hemophilia to attempt to be excused from a test or unwanted activity by feigning a bleed. He's probably not really lying or being manipulative; he's testing his limits and yours. It's a natural part of development and a golden opportunity to teach your child the consequences of his actions.

He may also cry wolf: if he craves your attention, and is too young to adequately verbalize his fears, he may inflate the symptoms of a real bleed or even imagine one.

How should you respond? Stress personal responsibility. His realization that he is different doesn't entitle him to invent bleeds or irresponsibly ignore them. He needs to learn to solve his problems, not use hemophilia to avoid them. He can be infused and still make up a class test, later that day or later that week. He can still attend gym class even if he's sidelined. He can complete classwork that his friends bring home.

A LITTLE HELP FROM HIS FRIENDS

At school, peers may contribute to your child's feeling different. He's surrounded by new children who enjoy competing, comparing, and boasting about possessions, families, and skills. He'll want to compete with them, to be liked and accepted. Hemophilia probably won't be noticeable, at least outwardly. On the other hand, when bleeds occur, your child can't hide the fact that he's different. The key to helping him gain acceptance is to be casual and honest, and keep it simple.

What should you tell other children about hemophilia, and who should tell them—you or your child? Generally, children are compassionate toward classmates when the situation is explained in terms they can understand. Explanations of hemophilia should not produce feelings of guilt or blame in your child.

If you prepare him well, you can leave it up to your child to tell his friends. Here's how you can help him:

- List only a few things that he should tell his classmates.
- Avoid crisis mode. Don't focus on worst-case scenarios.
- Emphasize what he can do! Minimize differences between him and his peers.
- Be relaxed and casual. Your attitude is contagious.

When you and your child are asked directly about hemophilia, don't respond for him. Let him respond, or wait until he's gone. If you answer for him, and he remains the silent third party, you discourage his independence. If you prepare him by rehearsing a response in advance, and then leave the explanation up to him, he'll feel confident and comfortable.

Having a close circle of friends is a great way for your child to gain stability if hemophilia gets rocky. True friends accept him unconditionally and make hemophilia seem like the minor difference it really is. Peers can show your child that everyone is different. He'll meet kids with disabilities, kids from single-parent and two-parent homes, and kids from different backgrounds. What a great opportunity to learn tolerance, acceptance, and community spirit!

BULLIES

There's one peer we all could probably do without: the bully. Bullies project their own feelings of anger, fear, or inadequacy onto someone they perceive as being weaker. Bullying means intimidating someone through physical behavior or verbal harassment. Depending on your child's demeanor and appearance, he may be perceived as being weaker, and he can become the target of bullying.

As a parent, you can intervene by contacting your child's teacher or the bully's parents, or by speaking to the bully yourself. Or you can empower your child to handle the bully. Share these important tips for dealing with bullies:

- Make your body language say, "I'm strong!" Head high, chin out, look confident.
- Use humor. "I guess I'm not worthy of fighting you, O great one!"
- Walk away. Hold your head high, refuse to fight, but don't run.
- Agree with the bully. Nothing so disarms a bully—child or adult!
- Scream or yell. Startle the bully with something unexpected.
- Use authority. When needed, ask an adult to intervene.[5]
- Stand up to the bully. Tell him you won't be pushed around!
- Ignore the bully. Pretend he doesn't exist.
- Use defensive physical action if attacked: block, duck, retreat.
- Try to make friends. Use the bully's name.[6]

Help your child understand why some children bully others: they may be influenced by violence in the media, or they may live in unhappy homes where violence is used as discipline. Bullies may only be seeking attention and approval from their peers. Your child will feel more competent and confident when he knows how to defend himself nonviolently. Sometimes confidence alone is enough to make the bully back off!

ACTIVITIES, ACCOMPLISHMENTS, AND EGO

Even bullies won't permanently damage a resilient child with strong self-esteem. Positive self-esteem is probably the chief factor in determining success in life. People with healthy self-esteem take responsibility for their actions and resist defeat. They feel capable, so they persevere.

Through their behavior and words, parents can encourage healthy self-esteem. How parents feel about and react to hemophilia is a major influence on their child's own attitude.

Because self-esteem is mostly learned, give your child the chance to discover what he's good at and what he can accomplish. Positive self-esteem grows from consistent and sincere recognition—by parents, teachers, and peers—of real accomplishments. Children need to hear more than "Oh, you're so smart," or "You look nice." They need specific compliments: "You built that model all by yourself? That's great!" Give generous praise, but be sure it is sincere and deserved.

What are your child's skills? What does he enjoy doing? Does he have special accomplishments, like doing a cartwheel or somersault? Did he win a ribbon at school, read a book by himself, or perform in a recital? Can he play an instrument? If you're unsure of his skills and can think of no concrete accomplishments, help him find an activity he does well and enjoys. Try classes in dance, art, music, crafts, or martial arts. He can learn to play the flute, build models, or take photographs. He can learn to fish or collect stamps. At ages six to twelve, children love collections. Marbles, bottle tops, superhero cards, gemstones, sporting cards, pennies—the list is endless! Help him start a collection and learn from it. Your child can become an expert, perhaps in an area where no other friend excels.

Activities with measurable outcomes—like trophies, ribbons, or karate belts earned—create feelings of success. Success will motivate your child because with each success, he builds self-esteem. He earned it!

Strategies for Building Self-Esteem

- Find appropriate activities for your child's age and skill level.
- Keep trying until you find something he does well and enjoys.
- Give specific compliments: "I love the colors you chose for that painting."
- Let him express his feelings, both positive and negative, about his activity.
- Avoid pressuring him into one activity or sport just because you enjoy it.
- Avoid pressure, such as "I know you can do it."
- Allow him to quit an activity if he gave it a good try.
- Avoid predicting what he will become based on his hobbies now: "You'll be an engineer because you're so good at building models!"
- Focus on his enjoyment and skills today: "You are really good at model building! I love how this model ship came out."

School Days
Chapter 10 Summary

- Starting school is a milestone. The world will now meet your child with hemophilia.
- Meet with school personnel before school starts. Ask your HTC nurse to attend.
- Provide some simple hemophilia books as an introduction. Try selecting three main points.
- Tell school personnel how to reach you at all times: provide phone numbers.
- Teachers should avoid overprotecting, singling out your child, denying hemophilia or bleeds, and overreacting.
- The school nurse is your first line of defense when seeking proper medical treatment for your child.
- If your child misses school, have homework emailed or brought home. Ask for a tutor.
- Your child may realize that he's different from his peers. He may start ignoring bleeds to fit in or crying wolf to draw attention.
- Teach your child about nonviolent ways to handle bullies.
- Build self-esteem by finding activities he does well and enjoys.

11

Sports and Summer Camp

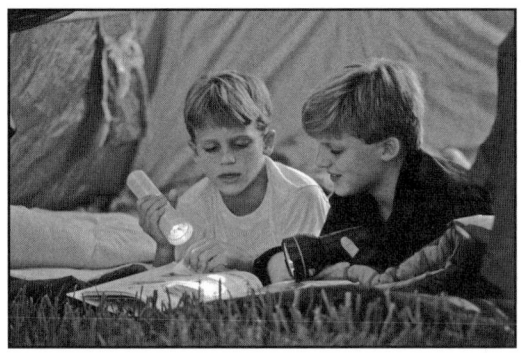

MacKale is such a typical boy. He has one speed—fast—and one volume—loud. He climbs, digs, runs, jumps, and we do little to prevent him from doing things that any normal boy loves to do. —Marsha M. Moffit McGuire, Michigan

Here are two great ways to encourage your child's independence and positive self-esteem: physical activity and summer camp. Physical activity is anything from walking to biking to organized sports. Although children with hemophilia shouldn't play contact sports like football, hockey, or boxing, no child—especially one with hemophilia—should be excluded from physical activities.

Physical activity helps children become skilled and accomplished. It's like chicken soup for self-esteem. Being active is also good for your child's physique and helps control bleeds. Strong muscles cushion blows and support joints. A lean body reduces stress on joints and makes finding veins easier. Good coordination improves your child's ability to avoid or handle trips, falls, and bumps. Second only to factor, physical activity is the best medicine for your child, and two great places to find it are in sports and at summer camp.

BOYS MUST BE BOYS

Physical activity is essential for growing boys. Through hundreds of thousands of years of biochemical evolution, males are neurologically hard-wired for competition, aggression, and physical risk-taking.[1] So boys need to move, take up space, burn off energy, and compete with each other. One appropriate way to meet these needs is to engage boys regularly in physical activities and sports.

But physical activity doesn't need to involve sports. Though some children with hemophilia enjoy organized sports, they aren't for everyone. Parents should focus instead on keeping children active, which is important for everyone. Physical activity can be as simple as walking the dog briskly around the block, or as involved as taking a day hike with the family.

Your job is to find the physical activity your child will enjoy and master. Choose an activity that challenges his body, improves his physique, and develops new skills. With proper preparation and training, physical activity can actually lower the risk of bleeds.

IS YOUR CHILD READY?

Before your child begins a regular physical activity, be sure it's appropriate for him. Have him examined by his regular physician and hematologist. Take him to an orthopedic specialist, who will check his joints and muscle coordination. Your hematologist knows your child's medical history, severity level, and trouble spots, and can help you make a good choice. If your child has a target joint or inhibitor, certain activities may be limited.

A toddler can participate in most normal childhood activities. Young children have supple joints, great flexibility, and boundless energy. Playgrounds without asphalt tops are ideal for developing bodies and increasing cognitive skills. Begin with swings, slides, and jungle gyms. Youngsters can start riding tricycles by age two, especially the "Big Wheel" style tricycles that are low to the ground. Introduce bicycles with training wheels at about age three. Give your child jump ropes and balls, take trips to the beach or pool, and get into the action yourself! Your child can begin team sports around age six. Even activities that seem risky, such as gymnastics, T-ball, or martial arts, aren't so risky when scaled down to a child's abilities.

THE DANGERS OF OBESITY

Your child is at greater risk of having joint problems if he doesn't exercise. Compounding this is the epidemic of obesity in America, which increases the risk of joint damage and bleeds. Everywhere you look, adults and even children are gaining weight at alarming rates. The CDC estimates that almost three-quarters of American adults aged 20 and older are overweight.[2] The United States has the highest obesity rate in the world.

Why are we now the fattest country on earth? Many factors contribute to obesity, and many are under our control—obesity is preventable. Two significant factors are lack of exercise (sedentary lifestyle) and poor diet (primarily fast food). Advanced technology has given us reason not to move. We spend lots of screen time in front of the television, video games, cell phones, and computers. Sedentary lifestyle is a major risk factor for obesity. And we consume well over $110 billion annually on fast food.[3] Most fast food is high in carbohydrates and fats and is often downed with sugary soft drinks, all of which pack a lot of calories, contributing to weight gain.

Obesity levels among children are skyrocketing. The CDC estimates that obesity rates have not changed since 2003: more than 12 million US children and adolescents aged 2 to 19 are obese, triple the number from just one generation earlier—and millions more are overweight.[4] Childhood obesity can lead to diabetes, high blood pressure, high cholesterol, and other conditions.

To safeguard your child's health, you must do more than just infuse factor. You must take a long, hard look in the mirror. Are you overweight? Is your child? If you have an infant with hemophilia, will you allow him to become overweight? How can you prevent it?

Being overweight or obese increases the risk of joint damage. A one-pound increase in weight results in four additional pounds of stress on the knee when walking. It's harder to find veins in an overweight child. Heavier children need more factor to control bleeds, possibly increasing your out-of-pocket costs. And overweight children are less likely to exercise, so they're at higher risk of joint bleeds.

As a responsible parent, you must assess the family's weight issues, create a plan with a physician, and make positive, permanent lifestyle changes. Throw away the soft drinks. Shut off the television and limit the gaming. Get outside with your child, daily if possible. Make physical activity into family time: join the YMCA, swim, walk, bike. Just a little every day is all it takes. You'll be amazed at the difference in your energy level, appetite control, food choices, mood—and waistline!

WHICH ACTIVITIES WILL YOUR CHILD CHOOSE?

As your child grows, he'll gravitate toward activities that appeal to him. Find an activity that he can do well, or simply enjoys, so he'll stick with it long enough to make progress and develop competence.

Consider your child's personality. Is he active and outgoing, maybe even hyper? Is he driven to compete? Is he coordinated? Does he love to climb? Can he focus and follow directions? Some children are natural athletes: coordinated, energetic, strong. Some are not overly physical, so finding the appropriate activity may be challenging. Some dislike organized sports, perhaps to their father's dismay, preferring to do activities on their own.

Your child can enroll in Little League if he likes team sports. He can enjoy activities oriented more toward the individual, such as swimming, weight lifting, bicycling, gymnastics, or martial arts. Swimming is highly recommended for children with hemophilia. Your child's enthusiasm will help you judge. Be patient. Many children balk at new activities, or their enthusiasm fizzles after a few months. Activity selection may take some bargaining: "Why not try this for two months? If you don't like it after that, you can try something else."

Your child's severity level may help determine the kinds of activities you consider, unless he is on prophylaxis. All sports carry some degree of risk, even for children without hemophilia. Having hemophilia may mean taking extra precautions and carefully weighing the risks versus benefits. Infuse prophylactically before strenuous physical activity, as a precaution.

PREPARATION

Physical activities are more fun when you feel prepared and know what to expect. Prepare your child for physical activity with physical conditioning and a review of rules and regulations.

Conditioning means slowly building up your child's fitness and ability level so he can successfully participate in an activity. Conditioning might involve some running, stretching, and lifting small weights. If your child is overweight, this will take time. Encourage small achievements, like walking around the block. Over time, his stamina and accomplishments will grow.

Your child should warm up before beginning any activity. Good conditioning helps your child do better and reduces the likelihood of injury. Stretching after exercising is also an essential part of any physical activity. The best person to teach you the correct way to stretch is your HTC physical therapist. The secret is to warm up before the activity and stretch consistently, after any activity.

Periodically review your child's personal responsibilities along with any sporting rules:

- Infusing before an activity, if necessary
- Knowing when his body has had enough
- Being able to diagnose a bleed during and after an activity

Remind him to tell you as soon as possible if he has a bleed. When he gets a bleed while participating in a sporting event, depending on your HTC instructions, he should

- infuse,
- elevate the affected area to keep blood flow moderated,
- ice the area, and
- rest.[5]

He should also have someone call you as soon as possible. These are big responsibilities that come with the privilege of playing a sport or activity.

Don't forget about regular safety rules! When you're teaching your child to ride a bicycle, explain bike safety rules: wear a helmet, ride in the same direction as traffic, and stop and look three times before crossing the street.[6] Remind him about standard playground rules: never go up a slide the wrong way, and be careful walking in front of a swing. Condition your child's behavior with rules and regulations while you condition his body for excellence.

GEAR UP!

Did you know that millions of teeth are knocked out each year during school sports activities such as basketball, baseball, and soccer? Yet only one-third of young athletes wear mouth guards!

You can reduce the risk of injury during activities by having your child wearing protective gear. Review with your child's coach or instructor the necessary protective devices and any optional devices. These include hard baseball helmets, protective cups, mouth guards, knee or elbow pads, chest pads, bicycle helmets, and wrist guards. Above all, make sure that these devices fit correctly. As your child grows, he'll need new protective gear.

MOVE IT!

> *Spencer is a member of the school track and soccer teams. In his off-season, he participates in skiing, bowling, ice skating, tennis, golf, and more. During the summer months, he and his father like to hang glide. With the exception of direct contact sports, we encourage Spencer to participate in all of life's activities.* —Andrea Brill, North Carolina

Being outdoors and moving isn't always a productive physical activity if you want to lose weight or get in shape. Walking the dog for 10 minutes or meandering along a beach is nice, but not enough. Long-lasting physical benefits require two types of exercise:

Cardio: overall body endurance movement like swimming, walking, bicycling, running, dancing
Strength training: using weights, resistance bands, or your own body weight

Cardio activities over 30 minutes raise your heart rate, helping to strengthen your most important muscle, your heart, for a more efficient body and longer life. Along with keeping your heart fit and your muscles toned, cardio keeps joints in good shape by reducing the frequency of joint bleeds.

Strength training involves resistance, pulling or pushing against something—even your own body weight—so that muscles contract and release. This helps them grow stronger. Strength training targets specific muscles. Strong muscles help protect joints. Your child can reduce his risk of joint bleeds when the muscles supporting his joints are strengthened.

NHF ranks physical activities according to safety level.[7] But along with safety, consider the health benefit of any activity. Golf is a low-risk sport often recommended for children with hemophilia. Golf is great, but it involves little resistance and even less aerobic activity. If your child loves golf, keep him at it, but make sure he has additional activities.

Swimming is the clear winner for best overall sport for children with hemophilia. It has no impact on joints, offers the highest aerobic benefit of any sport, and develops strong muscles that protect joints. Swimmers have the fewest joint bleeds, and fortunately, most children naturally love the water! Swimming can be a lifelong sport.

Once you select an activity, monitor it for competitiveness. What starts out as noncompetitive gymnastics—great for resistance and aerobics—may turn into a competitive, risky sport by the time your child enters high school. T-ball becomes baseball. Soccer games, with 55-pound eight-year-olds, become contests for 140-pound teens. When a sport or activity becomes so competitive that your teen risks serious injury, it's time to step back and reconsider. On the other hand, some individual sports, such as skiing, swimming, or running, can remain recreational through the years.

Choose activities and sports based on your child's condition, interest, and skills with a goal of improving aerobics and resistance. And get moving!

CAN'T? NO FOUR-LETTER WORDS ALLOWED!

At times, hemophilia means your child can't engage in physical activity. Target joints could signal the end of a baseball season. Inhibitors that don't respond to treatment could mean no team sports and limited physical activities. Surgery? Put the skateboard away for the summer. This can be hard on a child who sees his friends joining Little League or going mountain biking without him. But it doesn't mean he has to quit or feel defeated.

When the going gets tough, find a positive solution. Compensate for curtailed activities by finding something your child can do. If he can't play on an organized, competitive team, perhaps he can pursue his favorite activity off the team. He can play neighborhood kickball, tennis, or baseball with friends who understand his physical restrictions.

TAMING THE BARBARIAN

Sports may profoundly benefit self-esteem, with good coaching, equipment, and training. Physical activity, whether team or individual, builds expertise and skill, reinforcing a positive self-image. Children get concrete recognition for their achievements from coaches, teammates, and parents. Sports activities fulfill a child's need to be good at something.

Sports can also teach kids more advanced socialization skills. Children learn to work together and fit in when playing a team sport. They learn to follow and respect rules when competing with others. Team sports offer benefits that individual sports do not: working as part of a group, sharing defeats and victories, and depending on others. Children learn about getting hurt and setting limits for themselves.

Above all, sports provide an acceptable outlet for boys' natural impulses of aggression, high energy, and competition. If their aggression isn't channeled appropriately, they may find inappropriate outlets. They may bond with gangs instead of teammates; they may work out aggression through violence instead of physical activity. Through sports and physical activity, you can help your child with hemophilia overcome the feeling that he is different or weak. You can help him develop his sense of male identity by sharpening the skills and tendencies endowed by nature. You can also acknowledge that it's okay to be male—even if he still eats like a barbarian at the dinner table!

HEMOPHILIA SUMMER CAMP: LETTING GO

Hole-in-the-Wall Gang Camp in Connecticut is awesome! Camp has swimming, woodworking, arts and crafts, fishing, nature walks, and horseback riding. It has a dance and a stage night. The counselors and volunteers are really nice. I was afraid to leave home the first time I went, but after that first year, I loved it so much that I wasn't afraid anymore. Any kid who has not gone or is afraid of leaving home should give camp a try. Camp is a great place! —Tony DiChiara Jr., Massachusetts

Attending summer camp is an excellent way for your child to find physical activities that appeal to him in a supervised setting designed for children with hemophilia. He'll develop physical skill and build his self-esteem. Summer camp offers something that's hard for parents to provide at home: a chance to fly away from under your protective wing. For no matter how you try to grant your child freedom, your shadow is everywhere in his young life, and your relationship with him is probably intense. Being on their own, without parents to defer to or look up to, is a step toward maturity that most kids welcome.

It's normal for parents to be nervous about sending their child with hemophilia away for a week. It helps to know that qualified staff will be present—hemophilia nurses, trained counselors, and physical education coaches.

Camp is exciting, but it may also be intimidating for your child at first. Feeling separation anxiety is normal for any child, especially if he has depended on you for infusions. If your child is socially immature or particularly dependent, camp can help him mature.

How do you know if your child is ready for camp? Observe how he handles sleepovers. Is he homesick after only a few hours? Is he comfortable staying all night? Has he stayed with friends and neighbors as well as close relatives? If he handles sleepovers comfortably, he might be ready to try a bigger adventure.

11 Sports and Summer Camp

SELECTING A CAMP

All hemophilia summer camps are not created equal.[8] They have similarities and differences. Here's how they are alike:

- Each camp is staffed with a hemophilia nurse, and some have a social worker, physical therapist or doctor on staff.
- There are daily medical checks and infusions for injuries.
- Every camp teaches self-infusion—perhaps the main reason to send your child to camp.

Here's how they differ:

- Some camps are mixed, enrolling children with hemophilia and children with other blood disorders or disabilities.
- Some are solely for children with hemophilia.
- Some are for both boys and girls.
- Some allow families to stay, and some allow only siblings.
- Some are for specific age groups.
- Some provide extensive training for counselors, while others rely on untrained volunteers.

Each camp has its own philosophy. They all offer different activities.

Consider the following list before deciding on a camp for your child. If one camp doesn't meet your expectations, use these questions to find a camp that does.

- How long does camp last?
- Is camp only for children with hemophilia?
- Are the any costs?
- How is infusion taught?
- Which age groups will attend?
- Are families allowed to attend? Siblings?
- What training do counselors receive? Do they have hemophilia?
- Are there special events, such as overnight camping, river rafting, or talent shows?

- How is discipline handled? What rules are children expected to follow?
- How is homesickness handled? Can my child call home, or is this discouraged?
- What is the camp philosophy? Is there a religious, ethnic, or regional theme?
- What is the ratio of counselor to campers? Suggested ratios are 1:6 (one counselor to six campers) for ages 6 to 8; 1:8 for ages 9 to 14; 1:10 for ages 15 to 17.
- Who are the counselors? What is their training?
- Who are the medical staff? Can I meet them personally?
- What menu is offered? Can the camp accommodate special dietary needs?
- Which activities are offered?
- What are the protocols for medical emergencies?

Typical camp activities include archery, swimming, boating, volleyball, board games, ping-pong, tennis, tower climbs, hikes, nature walks, woodworking, crafts, and scavenger hunts. Some camps offer rock rappelling, whitewater rafting, and horseback riding. If your child is interested in a particular activity, find out if the camp offers it. If possible, visit the camp to get a feel for where your child will stay.

CAMPING OUT, GROWING UP

Your child may get plenty of physical activity at home or school. But camp gives him the unique experience of meeting other children his age with hemophilia. He may also meet young men or older adults with hemophilia who can serve as role models, demonstrating physical skill and positive self-esteem. Because many counselors attend camp as volunteers, their devotion often indicates strong self-esteem and the desire to pass on this quality to the next generation.

Your child will benefit from meeting other children like him. This may be the first time he's ever seen other kids and adults with hemophilia. He may become less egocentric, less isolated, and more independent. He'll be part of a tribe, a group where he especially belongs that accepts him unconditionally. He'll receive much-needed recognition for his achievements—from adults other than you and his classroom teacher. Camp staff will reward and praise him for taking care of himself, infusing himself (if he is capable), and participating in camp activities. Counselors will be his mentors and role models, helping him develop confidence and a strong personal identity.

LEARNING SELF-INFUSION AT CAMP

One main purpose of camp is to foster independence through self-infusion. Self-infusion can be taught to children aged five and up, depending on the child's maturity and ease of venous access. A child with severe hemophilia or who has frequent infusions might be ready to learn sooner. A child with mild or moderate hemophilia may not be ready until after age 10 because he lacks experience with infusions. Many children come to camp able to perform all the infusion steps except the final one: the actual needlestick.

Successful self-infusion doesn't necessarily mean accurate self-diagnosis. Even if your child can physically follow the steps to infuse himself, it may be a long time before he can diagnose a bleed or respect that he needs an infusion. Boys often ignore pain if they're distracted throughout the day.

Your HTC nurse or hematologist can help you decide the best age for your child to begin self-infusion. These professionals can instruct him at the HTC. You can also wait until summer camp, where he'll be in a relaxed, happy, natural environment, surrounded by other children learning self-infusion. He'll probably receive an award when he learns, and can bask in the attention of other campers and counselors. Along with the talent show, climbing wall, swimming, and archery, his success in self-infusion may be the best achievement he brings home from camp!

Sports and Summer Camp
Chapter 11 Summary

- Physical activities, including sports, promote self-esteem, strong physique, and healthier joints.
- Prepare your child for physical activity with conditioning and a review of rules and regulations.
- Reduce injuries by having your child wearing protective gear that fits correctly.
- A good activity program requires both cardio and strength training.
- When certain sports, or all sports, are prohibited, find something physical your child can do.
- Summer camp offers physical activities in a supervised setting.
- Screen the camp. Ask specific questions about the program, camp location and facilities, staff, staff training and mission.
- Camp promotes socialization with other children who have hemophilia. Young adults or older men with hemophilia can serve as role models.
- Camp fosters independence by offering classes on self-infusion.

12

Family Matters

My older son, Mark, learned what was valuable in life by age five. He educated many adults, saying, "Now, is it really that important that you had a flat tire? At least your little brother isn't in the hospital right now because he is bleeding. Which is more important?" He has a tremendous sense of compassion, and he goes out of his way to help someone who is handicapped or ill or a child who is shunned. He is extremely aware of children with special needs and is always teaching people how to help these children.
—Anonymous

Hemophilia most directly affects you and your child with the disorder, but its emotional impact spreads to your extended family: siblings, grandparents, aunts, uncles, cousins. Hearing the diagnosis, family members may react with feelings that range from uncertainty, curiosity, or acceptance to disappointment, depression, or blame. These are all common and normal reactions.

After the diagnosis, you may need to focus on your immediate family first, helping siblings cope with the sudden attention given to a new baby with a medical condition. Soon, you'll also have to help your extended family. Although you may think of them as your support system and yourself as the person who needs support, your family will probably need your support and guidance. How can you help them when you are also just learning to cope? Fortunately, there are some things you can do to support your family, maintain boundaries when it gets intense, and still nurture everyone through this challenging time.

SIBLINGS: YOUR CHILDREN WITHOUT HEMOPHILIA

When Vivian Alexis was three, she didn't like the fact that her brothers got lollipops after infusions, and she did not. Sometimes she'd say that she had a bleed, for attention. —Erica Boone, Michigan

Siblings can be a wonderful source of companionship, comfort, and fun! We've all witnessed deep compassion between siblings when one has a medical condition. Yet it's normal for children to feel curious, jealous, ignored, or even hostile when a sibling has a chronic illness. Siblings see their parents' intense concern for the child with hemophilia: their brother may be allowed special privileges, such as skipping school or chores because of a bleed. Or he may get extra attention from relatives and neighbors. Perceiving discrepancies in attention and treatment, siblings without hemophilia may have negative feelings.

Young children can't often name or verbalize their feelings. Emotions are expressed as whines, complaints, tantrums, or misbehavior. Much of this is simply a cry for attention from Mom or Dad. Right or wrong, children perceive that their needs are not being met. Sibling rivalry is often a way of saying, "I need more attention."

When children believe their needs are being met, behavior usually calms down, and they regain emotional control. You can address your children's needs in many ways, but it's crucial to give your children a sense of worth—by meeting their unique needs, spending time alone with them, and acknowledging their feelings.

TREAT EACH CHILD UNIQUELY

It's impossible to treat your children equally. And children don't want to be treated equally. Children are not equal. Each child has specific needs, exclusive talents, unique beliefs, varied expectations, and distinct developmental patterns. Yet in an effort to show our children that we love them equally, we often try to treat them equally.

"You love him more than me!" "Why did you buy him something and not me?" "Why did he get two lollipops, and I only have one?" These questions show that your child is trying to assess self-worth by comparing himself to his sibling. Avoid giving in to demands, treating each child exactly the same, or comparing each child's needs. Instead, redirect the question or statement to meet your child's individual needs:

"I do spend a lot of time with your brother because he needs me. But what can you and I do together when I'm finished?"

"I bought him a present because he was extra patient at the hospital for his infusion. Anyone in this family who achieves something is rewarded, and that includes you."

"He received two lollipops because he asked for two. If you want two, you may have two."

These examples successfully address the comment or question separately from the need; any comparison to the sibling is broken. When you focus on children's individual needs, without comparing them to their siblings, you attend to the true, core issue. What's the core issue? It might be reassurance of worth, fear of abandonment, need for attention, or the desire to be heard.

To find your children's unique needs, enlist their help! Invite them to talk to you: "Would you like to tell me the best thing that happened to you today?" Talk about the things your children find special, which usually involve a parent: reading a book before bedtime, going out for a treat, or perhaps choosing the night a child gets to sleep in Mom and Dad's bed.

Don't make negative comparisons between your children out loud. This can diminish each sibling's individuality and breed resentment. Avoid saying things like this:

"Your brother never cries when he gets his shot."

"Why can't you be more like your sister?"

"You're going to make everyone late because you won't help with this infusion!"

"Of all the kids, you are the slowest!"

"Of all the kids, you are the smartest!"

Even so-called positive comments, like the last one, make your child look good only when compared to someone who doesn't look quite so good. This can hurt the relationship between siblings. Instead, identify and praise each child's special skill, and acknowledge his or her unique needs, with no comparison to anyone else:

"I can tell that fall hurt you because you're crying. I'm glad you came to me so I can help."

"Do you want to read a book now? Let me finish this infusion first, and in about fifteen minutes, I would love to read you that book!"

"As soon as I finish speaking to Johnny's doctor and see if I need to give him an infusion, you and I can make some cookies and then eat them all up! Sound good?"

Although you treat each child uniquely, don't forget to voice the expectation that children follow common family rules. Except when a bleed prevents it, don't excuse the child with hemophilia from family rules concerning chores or conduct because of his condition, or because of your guilt or sadness. If one sibling tantrums for attention, don't allow that child to escape disciplinary consequences if you normally apply them. Treat children uniquely, but also treat them fairly.

SPEND TIME WITH EACH CHILD

When you value something, you spend time with it. From toddlers to adolescents, children often equate love with the amount of time a parent spends with them. When one sibling sees you spending extra time with the child with hemophilia—hovering, warning, monitoring, or just gasping—you may appear to be more interested in that child. The sibling without hemophilia may feel less loved. Ultimately, children want to know, "Am I special? Do you consider me worthy enough to spend time with? To worry about?"

Every child needs attention. Giving enough attention to meet a child's needs may require lots of time. It's challenging, isn't it? Each child needs time, but the child with hemophilia may need even more time. You also need time to nurture yourself and enjoy relationships with others.

Even if time is limited or you are rushed, you can provide brief but constant reassurance throughout the day, reminding your child you will have time later on.

- Give your child frequent hugs and kisses.
- Create a special signal, unique to your child, to show affection.
- Address your child with a special nickname.
- Tell your child you've set aside time to spend together later.
- Let your child choose a favorite activity to share later.

This last suggestion is useful when regular routine is disrupted. Daily routines give children a sense of security, and disruption may cause stress. For example, if bedtime stories are interrupted, relieve some stress by showing that you haven't forgotten the routine. Tell your child that although you can't read a story because you're taking her brother to the hospital, you'll read two extra stories the next night. Sometimes, just acknowledging that there is a routine is enough to reassure the sibling.

Involve your children without hemophilia in their sibling's care. When children are involved, they feel useful and needed instead of helpless and unimportant. Assign them specific responsibilities, such as getting the factor ready or applying the tourniquet. They may feel less resentful when they know they're needed. They can spend special time with you, doing a special job.

ACKNOWLEDGE SIBLINGS' FEELINGS

"Be nice to your brother. He has hemophilia!" Have you ever heard yourself say this? Or have you heard your child without hemophilia say, "I'm glad he has hemophilia so he gets a shot. He's mean to me!"

Negative feelings are common for siblings, and not altogether unhealthy. What matters is how you handle feelings, and how you teach your children to handle them. If negative feelings are constantly squelched, siblings begin to think, "Mom and Dad love me only when I'm nice to my brother and don't get mad." If you ignore or downplay your child's negative feelings, you invalidate them. The child then believes that some feelings aren't important. In truth, it's normal and acceptable not to like a family member sometimes!

Remember: An acknowledgment is not an endorsement of the feeling. It's an endorsement of the child. You are not saying, "It's okay to hate your brother." You're saying, "It's okay to feel like you hate your brother sometimes." Acknowledging tells children that their feelings are important and that they are important. Once you acknowledge feelings, you can move toward coping with them positively.

Give siblings a vote of confidence by stepping back and letting them work out a conflict. This usually works with children aged four and older, and when you monitor close by. Try not to referee a conflict by ending it, making judgments, or providing a solution. Children need to learn to find solutions for themselves. When two children want to use the same toy, listen in and observe, but don't intrude. See how they approach the problem.

You might be able to prevent problems by reminding children, when not involved in competitive play or discussion, about the rules you have established to respect each other's feelings: "Here are the toys you wanted. Try to remember to ask when you want a toy. We don't grab for toys without asking." And remember that you are modeling appropriate interactions daily. Your children watch how you successfully, joyfully, and respectfully communicate with friends, neighbors, teachers, and family members.

> **Validate Your Child's Feelings**
>
> - Lovingly verbalize your child's feelings: "You seem angry."
> - Tell your child that it's okay to have negative feelings.
> - Tell your child that it's not okay to use negative feelings to hurt someone, either inside (emotionally) or outside (physically).
> - Avoid rushing to fix the situation. Wait, be quiet, and see how your children handle it.
> - Don't immediately judge what you see: "You two are being bad!" Instead, first describe what you see: "I see two kids who are really mad at each other!" Let your children make the next move, as long as it's nonviolent.
> - Don't tell your children how they should feel. Avoid saying things like, "Never hate your sister!" "Don't be angry!" "You should appreciate the outfit your aunt gave you."
> - Set behavior limits with consequences. "We do not allow hitting. Two minutes in time out."
> - Allow children to express negative feelings without judging. Avoid saying, "You're naughty to say you don't like your brother!"

TEACH SIBLINGS ABOUT HEMOPHILIA

One way to help your children without hemophilia cope is to teach them about hemophilia in an age-appropriate way. The more they learn, the more they'll understand why hemophilia takes up so much of your time. Beginning at age three or four, your children can learn about hemophilia in concrete terms: "When your brother gets hurt, he needs medicine to get better." Or if the sibling is on prophylaxis: "Your brother gets a shot to stay healthy." By the time your children enter school, you can give more complicated explanations, including what's missing from their sibling's blood, how joints and muscles bleed, and how factor makes it better.[1]

Children of different ages need different explanations. Instead of gathering your family together to offer one explanation, find time to spend with each child individually. Tailor your explanations appropriately, based on the child's age, and respond to every question.

Preschool siblings may blame themselves for causing bleeds. Because preschoolers are egocentric, they believe they're the cause of many events in their small worlds. When the child with hemophilia is hurt, it's natural for parents to ask, "What did you do to him?" Then, of course, siblings may blame themselves. Try to avoid assigning blame.

Preschoolers, obsessed with good and bad, may fear "catching" hemophilia as a result of negative feelings toward their sibling. As sisters get older, they may wonder whether they are carriers and will eventually bear children with hemophilia. When a child with hemophilia is in pain, siblings may even feel guilty that he has hemophilia and they don't. You can ease many negative feelings if you spend time with each child, listening without judging, providing information according to age, and offering attention based on need.

And it's not all negative! Your child with hemophilia has so much to offer his siblings. The whole family can learn lessons in patience,

12 Family Matters

tolerance, independence, respect, and compassion. When your children without hemophilia learn to manage powerful feelings about a sibling, they develop a sense that they're in charge of their lives.

WHAT GRANDPARENTS, AUNTS, AND UNCLES SHOULD KNOW

Relatives can be a vital source of support during your first few years with hemophilia. A sister who listens, a mother who comes in a pinch to watch your children while you visit the clinic, a father who offers to take his grandchild with hemophilia fishing, and most valued of all, relatives who call to say, "How can I help?" These people bring normalcy, humor, support, and perspective.

And yet, aren't relatives often the ones who drive us crazy? Although hemophilia can be a big shock to every family member, in some ways it's even harder for those who don't live with it every day. Your relatives' reactions may closely mirror your own stages of acceptance: denial, anger, and grief. Unfortunately for you, because they don't live with hemophilia daily and may live far away, some family members may never resolve their initial feelings. They may always seem to be stuck in a stage. Relatives strain your relationship when they are perpetually depressed over hemophilia, constantly fear bleeds, or remind you frequently that you gave your child hemophilia.

Even when hemophilia is known to run in a family, everyone hopes that the odds will be favorable. When those hopes are crushed, relatives may react with drama as if it's the first time hemophilia has appeared in the lineage!

At the core of any family member's undesirable reaction is *fear*— fear that something terrible will happen to the baby, fear of the unknown, fear of being unable to prevent bleeds. Your relatives love your child and naturally fear for him. They also love you. But sometimes fear expresses itself in excessive control or visible anxiety, rather than in gentle communication and honest feelings. Relatives may exhibit blame, shame, guilt, denial, overprotection, or rigidity. Fear may create an overbearing in-law who enforces strict house rules when you visit, and won't allow your child to act with normal spontaneity or energy. Fear may create an aunt who audibly gasps whenever your child runs or falls. Fear may be at the root of the interrogation you receive after an accident: "*Why* didn't you have his safety belt on?" "Why do you *let* him jump off the bed?" "Why did you expose him to that unnecessary CT scan?"

Some families are proud of being from "healthy" stock, and view people who consult doctors as hypochondriacs or physically weak. Hemophilia shatters this family belief and creates a fear of vulnerability. As they desperately seek an explanation, it's common for such families to offer magical or religious solutions in the hope of curing a child. To them, this was simply not supposed to happen.

When hemophilia is known to run in the family, relatives may fear that they could have a child with hemophilia themselves. Or they may feel guilty that they might have helped contribute to hemophilia's inheritance. With all these simmering emotions, you may need some strategies to maintain emotional boundaries and family peace.

HOW TO HANDLE UNWANTED ADVICE AND COMMENTS

My side of the family has never had any issues, as we are very familiar with hemophilia. But my husband's side is a different story. They have no desire to learn about it. They don't understand hemophilia and the problems associated with it. When he needs rest in order to recover from a bleed, we are "babying him." If he gets injured in school and needs to come home for a treatment, we are being "overprotective." This is very frustrating, even though I am constantly trying to educate them. —Deborah Murray, New York

12 Family Matters

That's right: your family members may not behave as you wish. This is a letdown at first, especially if you need support. And it challenges the belief that if you just try hard enough, you can change others—like your relatives. Truthfully, the only person you can really change is *you*. How?

- You can learn to manage your responses and tone down your reactions.
- You can avoid acting defensively or resentfully, which may only escalate tension and alienation.
- You can help your family cope positively with hemophilia
- You can avoid making hemophilia the battlefield of your relationship.

Realize that when relatives criticize, blame, or judge, it's often because of their own fear or discomfort, not because of hemophilia or because of you. So don't take it as a personal attack! Try not to be defensive. Don't explain, blame, or apologize. To end the downward spiral of negativity, try the tactics listed here. You may be able to preserve the relationship by redefining it.

Restate kindly what relatives say. "You think that Kyle should wear a helmet all the time?" or "You believe that I gave this to him?" This often defuses a tense situation because you are responding, not reacting.

Make a statement about your feelings, not theirs. Start your statement with *I*. "I believe . . ." "I feel that . . ." "I think . . ." (No, "I think you're wrong" doesn't count!) "I feel confident that I'm a good parent and can handle this." "I believe deciding to have more children is a personal decision between the parents." Avoid *You* statements: "You shouldn't be so worried all the time about my son." "You make me angry when you keep harping on how he shouldn't play ball!" Statements beginning with *I* express and define the self, but *You* statements accuse or blame. Blame and accusation destroy communication and understanding.

Offer nonjudgmental comments that acknowledge the other person's opinion and discomfort. Nothing can take the wind out of someone's sails like saying, "That's an interesting way to look at it," instead of, "Why don't you keep your opinions to yourself?" Or try, "Yes, it's very possible that he might get hurt." "I sense that you're worried, and I appreciate that." "Yes, his port does make him stand out at the pool." "I suppose sometimes we are a little overprotective." "You could be right." You are not agreeing with what the other person said; you are simply acknowledging the person's opinions and feelings.

Don't use your family as your only means of emotional support. Find some support in a less intense relationship. Your HTC and local hemophilia organization probably have support groups to help parents and families cope.

Use humor! Nothing defuses a conflict like well-timed humor. When relatives comment negatively on your child's numerous colorful bruises, reply with a smile, "But I like the moldy cheese look!" Say to nervous onlookers, "After this infusion, don't give him any juice; we don't want him sprouting a leak!"

Your HTC can help with especially stubborn family members. HTC social workers often volunteer to meet with family members. Some relatives argue every medical decision made by your child's team. Ask if your doctor is willing to talk to aggressive family members. This removes you from the line of fire, so you aren't hit with everyone's raw emotions.

Don't forget that families can be a source of great comfort. Perhaps because they don't live so closely with hemophilia, they can offer perspective and relief. If you have relatives who give you the help you need, you're fortunate! If you don't, you have a golden opportunity to forge a new relationship with them by examining, and then changing, your own responses to explosive or unproductive situations.

12 Family Matters

TIPS FOR RELATIVES

Ask me whatever questions you have! Your interest and concern help me. Your fear and silence destroy me. —Pat Russomano, New Jersey

Your relatives love your child and want to help. But how? How can they be supportive but not intrusive? Should they talk openly about hemophilia? Should they act like nothing has happened? Should they express their fears? Help your relatives respond appropriately and constructively by giving them guidelines, modeling appropriate behavior, or reminding them gently. The following recommendations for family members come from other parents of children with hemophilia. Consider sharing them with your own family.

Treat the child with hemophilia normally. As an important adult in this child's life, don't say he is different, unhealthy, or cursed. Don't overprotect or coddle him. Try not to gasp or moan, "Poor child!" Project a positive attitude to help him develop a good self-image. Focus on what he can do, not on what he can't do.

Show concern but not pity. Pity makes a child feel self-conscious, aware that something is "wrong" with him. Pity emphasizes our differences. Stress the positive. Show your young relative compassion about a particular injury, but don't pity him.

Ask for advice. Parents will gladly suggest ways to be positive, and will explain to you what their child can do. Be willing to accept the parents' standards of care, even if you think they're unnecessarily protective or lenient.

Learn about hemophilia. The more you learn about hemophilia, the easier it becomes to treat your young relative normally. When you ask to learn more, you show your family that you care and that you appreciate what the family must cope with.

Don't judge. The family with hemophilia needs loving support, not advice or condemnation. Don't judge the decision to let the child play a sport, miss school, or attend school, or the decision to have another child.

Attend a support group meeting with the parents. There are even support groups specifically for relatives!

Learn to participate in the infusion process. As a relative, you can give tremendous relief to parents by learning the infusion process. Learn how to prepare factor, or, if you're brave, get trained to give the infusion. You'll become a safety net in a crisis, and can babysit your little relative with hemophilia!

Express concern and show interest. Parents need to talk about their ability to confront and overcome hemophilia. It's strange that some relatives complain about how hard it is to toilet train their two-year-old, but don't give the parents of a child with hemophilia the chance to describe how they successfully learned to do home infusions.

Acknowledge hemophilia in the child. Hemophilia is an integral part of your young relative's mental and physical being. Ignoring it means ignoring one of the most important things in his life.

As a relative, you're in a unique position to promote and reinforce a child's healthy self-image. It's one thing for parents to treat a child with hemophilia normally and casually, because they live with it. But you play a role that no one else can play. When a favorite uncle, cousin, or grandparent reinforces the message, "You are normal. You are loved unconditionally," the child's feeling of self-worth can light him up like fireworks!

Meeting Siblings' Needs

> After Zack was diagnosed, I tried hard to remain sensitive to my daughter Leah's physical and emotional needs, but the first few years were still difficult. Leah is six years older than Zack, so she was already independent and able to verbalize her feelings. Yet at times, she felt short-changed by her brother's medical problems. She also tended to suppress her feelings, which then manifested in physical complaints such as stomachaches, headaches, and minor injuries that "needed" our attention. Once Leah told me that she understood why Zack's bleeds were much more serious than her own illnesses or injuries, but she felt that we didn't pay as much attention to her problems. I told her that I understood her feelings, and I apologized for not taking more time to tend to her needs.
>
> I had our pediatrician evaluate Leah's stomachaches, and I even started wrapping her "injuries" with the same bandages her brother used. Just having more of my undivided attention, along with the physical "proof" that she got hurt, too, or needed to see a doctor is what helped Leah get through this phase quickly.
>
> To prevent Leah from believing that she needed to be injured or ill to get attention, we scheduled special dates. A simple shopping trip, lunch, or a movie was easy to do. Just taking the time to talk together without being interrupted also helped. We gave Leah choices about helping with Zack's home infusions, participating in our local foundation events, and attending summer camp.
>
> Leah has gained so much compassion, self-confidence, and inner strength through this journey. The same is true for our entire family because we sought outside help when necessary, and we learned to work well together. Paying attention to siblings is important. After all, they're the ones who will raise their own children, and some will do so with an inherited bleeding disorder in the next generation.
> —Stephanie Dansker, California

Family Matters
Chapter 12 Summary

- Hemophilia affects the entire family, including siblings and relatives.
- It's normal for children to feel curious, jealous, ignored, or even hostile when a sibling has a chronic illness.
- Negative feelings or behavior are often a cry for parental attention.
- Address needs by treating each child uniquely, spending time alone together, and acknowledging feelings.
- Include the siblings without hemophilia in caring for the child with hemophilia.
- Some relatives may mask fear or anxiety about hemophilia by blaming, shaming, assigning guilt, or ignoring.
- Avoid being defensive: don't apologize, try to explain yourself, or justify your behavior or decisions when it makes you uncomfortable or angry.
- Make *I* statements, not *You* statements.
- Acknowledge the opinions and discomfort of others: "You could be right."
- Get support when you need it. You can find support outside your family at your local HTC or hemophilia organization.

13

Deciding to Have More Children

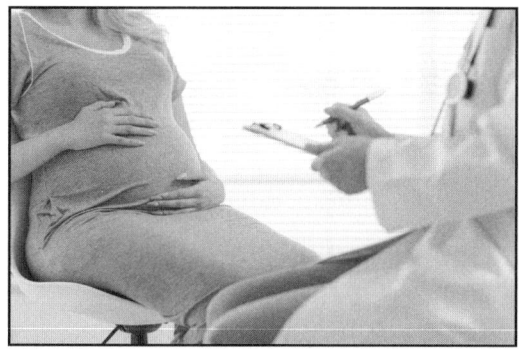

My father had hemophilia, so I knew I was a carrier. My husband and I received counseling before conceiving Stephen. The people at the HTC were so positive—they made us feel that we would be blessed to have a child with hemophilia. When I asked our nurse if she would ever advise a carrier against having children with hemophilia, she was speechless. She couldn't seem to find strong enough words to tell us how special these children are. Of course, now that we have Stephen, we agree. We wouldn't trade him for anything in the world! —Annamarie Asher, Michigan

Most couples dream of starting a family. You may one day stare longingly at other people's infants, and realize you're ready for your own child. You pore through books on baby names. You're overjoyed to learn you are pregnant. And when the happy day arrives, your dream of a new family has been fulfilled.

But the hemophilia diagnosis shatters your dream. You didn't count on something being wrong. And you may start wondering about future children. Should you have more? If your child with hemophilia is your second or third born, the decision to have more children might be irrelevant. If your child with hemophilia is your first born, then deciding to have more children might seem out of the question, or worrisome, or might be the last thing on your mind.

The decision to have more children is intensely personal. If hemophilia runs in your family, you may feel comfortable taking chances because you know what it's like to live with hemophilia; or you may decide not to have biological children. If you've had one child with hemophilia, perhaps you want to devote your time and financial resources to him—or you may find hemophilia so manageable that you can't wait to have another child.

Having more children is your decision. But first, learn about your options to determine your carrier status and whether your child has hemophilia. Then, if you know you are a carrier and decide to have children, you can plan for the birth. This chapter will explore these considerations to help you gain perspective.

WHAT IS A CARRIER?

The first step in family planning is to determine your carrier status. As discussed in Chapter 2, the X and Y chromosomes are called the sex chromosomes: males are created by the XY sex chromosome pairing and females by the XX. A carrier is a woman who has an X chromosome containing a defective gene for a clotting factor, which we call the hemophilia gene. She also has one X chromosome with a normal gene for clotting factor. Having an affected X chromosome means that each of her sons has a 50% chance of having hemophilia.

Having the hemophilia gene may also affect the factor level of the carrier. The X chromosome containing the hemophilia gene causes the body to produce little or no functional factor. But the unaffected X chromosome has a functional gene that allows for low to normal factor production, typically with factor levels of 40% to 80%. So, in some cases, a carrier may show no symptoms of hemophilia and may have normal or near-normal blood-clotting ability.

Can carriers show signs and symptoms of hemophilia? Yes! Women who have factor levels between 40% and 60% of normal have an increased risk of bleeding.[1] The lower the factor level, the greater the risk of bleeding. If a carrier's levels are below 50%, she actually has mild hemophilia. All women who are carriers, or suspected of being a carrier, should have their factor levels checked. If their levels are low, they should have a plan in place to treat bleeding in the event of trauma, heavy bleeding during menstruation, or other bleeding-related situations, such as childbirth.

ARE YOU A CARRIER?

Knowing that you *are not* a carrier simplifies the decision to have more children, because none of your children will be born with hemophilia. Knowing that you are a carrier will help you decide whether to get pregnant and help you plan for your pregnancy. Simple genetics can determine whether you are an **obligate** or **possible** carrier.

You are an obligate carrier (meaning you definitely carry the hemophilia gene) if *any one* of these conditions is true:

- Your father had hemophilia and you are female.
- You're the mother of more than one child with hemophilia.
- You're a mother who has one child with hemophilia and another biological relative with hemophilia.

You are a possible carrier if *either one* of these conditions is true:

- You are the mother of one child with hemophilia, and your family has no history of hemophilia.
- You have a female relative who is a carrier.

If you're a possible carrier, you may want to consider genetic testing,

- to positively identify your carrier status,
- to determine the chances of having children with hemophilia, and
- to prepare for the birth of a child with hemophilia.

If you're an obligate or possible carrier, visit the geneticist and social worker at an HTC for help in making family planning decisions. The social worker can help you fully understand how genetic testing options may affect your family planning decisions.

When you know you're a carrier, your chances of having a child with hemophilia are easy to calculate. The following will be true for every pregnancy:

- If you have a boy, there is a 50% chance that he will have hemophilia.
- If you have a girl, there is a 50% chance that she will be a carrier (see Chapter 2).

If you want to have biological children and would never terminate a pregnancy based on a prenatal diagnosis of hemophilia, then testing can help you make birthing decisions such as choosing the safest delivery method and having additional medical staff present who are knowledgeable about hemophilia. If you do not want a baby with hemophilia under any circumstance, then knowing you're a carrier may lead you to decide not to have biological children; you might consider adoption.

If you want a genetic test to determine your carrier status, arrange for the test long before you become pregnant. Genetic testing often involves a long wait for results, anywhere from a few weeks to a few months. If you have a male relative with hemophilia who can be tested, the specific mutation causing hemophilia can be determined, and your test results can arrive sooner, because the lab will be testing only for this specific mutation.

You can also test your daughter for carrier status. Your HTC can help you decide when and how to test her. The genetic counseling team will take into account her age, emotional maturity, anxiety level, and ability to handle the diagnosis. The team will assess the amount of information she already understands, and will offer further counseling to help her accept her test results. It's also important to have your

13 Deciding to Have More Children

daughter's factor level tested, especially if she shows signs of mild hemophilia: easy bruising; frequent nosebleeds; prolonged bleeding after tooth extractions; and, as a teen, prolonged or heavy menstrual periods. Be sure to have her tested before any surgery.

CARRIER TESTS

There are three basic methods of testing carrier status:

- Measurement of factor VIII or factor IX levels
- **Direct DNA** mutational analysis
- **Indirect DNA** linkage analysis

All three tests require blood samples for analysis.

Measurement of Factor Levels

Measuring a woman's factor VIII or IX levels is a screening test: low factor VIII or IX levels are a good indicator that she is a hemophilia carrier, but they aren't conclusive. A woman can be a carrier and still have low-normal to normal factor levels. The normal factor range is 50% to 150%. Carriers can show wide variation in factor levels: from almost no factor to high-normal factor levels. In general, the lower your factor VIII level, the greater the odds that you're a carrier, especially if your level is lower than 50%.[2]

If you're planning to have more children and your factor levels are not low, you need more accurate DNA testing, such as direct DNA mutational and indirect DNA linkage tests. Direct analysis searches your DNA for specific mutations of the factor VIII gene that are known to cause hemophilia. Indirect linkage analysis compares the DNA of your relatives, with and without hemophilia, to your own DNA.

Direct DNA Mutational Analysis

The direct DNA test is the most accurate way to determine your carrier status. This test uses a process called *DNA sequencing* to first examine the DNA of a family member with hemophilia—your child with hemophilia, or a brother, uncle, or grandparent. Doctors then compare your relative's DNA to a large data bank of known mutations in factor genes, gleaned from many carriers and people with hemophilia.[3] It may be possible to identify the exact location and nature of the mutation that causes hemophilia in your family. If a match is found between an affected family member and the data bank, then you can easily have your DNA tested to see if it contains the same mutation.

Direct testing is precise. If the tested DNA contains a recognized mutation, the woman is a carrier. If the mutation causing hemophilia in the woman's family is not present in the woman's DNA, she is not a carrier. One drawback: if you don't have a family member with hemophilia to test, or if doctors can't identify the mutation causing hemophilia in your family, it may be difficult or impossible to determine your carrier status using the direct test.

Indirect DNA Linkage Analysis

If the direct test can't determine your carrier status, your geneticist may suggest the indirect test.[4] First, DNA samples are taken from you and several family members, with and without hemophilia. The test compares the DNA samples to detect patterns that differ for affected versus unaffected family members. These differences can then be used as markers for hemophilia. Once markers have been identified, the test then looks at whether your DNA resembles the affected or unaffected members. If it resembles the affected family members, this strongly indicates that you are a carrier.

Indirect DNA analysis is accurate more than 90% of the time, assuming markers can be identified that distinguish affected from unaffected family members. When indirect tests fail to identify useful markers, the results are inconclusive.

Learning your carrier status opens many doors. You'll have choices to make, but your new knowledge may offer peace of mind and a sense of control over your future.

SYMPTOMATIC BLEEDING

If you're a carrier, you might have some bleeding problems of your own. Because you have one X chromosome that carries a functional gene for factor and one that carries the defective gene, the functional gene can't always produce factor for you at adequate levels. Some carriers' factor levels are less than 50%. These women risk excessive bleeding during dental extraction, surgery, trauma, and sometimes childbirth or post-childbirth. They may also have frequent nosebleeds, bruising, and heavy menstrual bleeding.

These women are called **symptomatic carriers** and can experience prolonged bleeding in certain situations, similar to men with mild hemophilia. But unlike males with mild hemophilia, symptomatic carriers have additional concerns. Some suffer from *menorrhagia*—heavy bleeding during a menstrual period or prolonged menstrual bleeding, lasting more than seven days. Others may have painful menstruation, or may bleed between menstrual periods.

Symptomatic carriers essentially have mild hemophilia. True! If they have bleeds, they are treated just like anyone with mild hemophilia. For those with factor VIII deficiency, treatment might include desmopressin or factor replacement therapy. For menorrhagia, treatment might include hormones or drugs affecting hormones, to reduce bleeding.

Desmopressin is a synthetic hormone that triggers the release of stored factor VIII into the bloodstream. Desmopressin can be used only once or twice during a 48-hour period, because once the body's reserves of factor VIII are depleted, it takes several days to replenish them. To use desmopressin, your factor level must be greater than 5% (the higher the better). Also, not all people respond the same way to desmopressin. Your hematologist may want to perform a desmopressin challenge test, in which you are given a dose of desmopressin and your factor levels are tested to determine how much they rise after the drug is given. For longer-term therapy or severe bleeds, factor replacement therapy may be needed.[5]

If you're a symptomatic carrier, get a baseline factor level test from your HTC. For hemophilia A carriers, this should be done before pregnancy, as factor VIII can rise 200% to 500% during pregnancy. Hemophilia B carriers don't see a rise in factor levels during pregnancy. Be aware, too, that although factor VIII levels increase during pregnancy, they drop off rapidly after birth, so the mother may be at risk of postpartum hemorrhaging or bleeding after cesarean section (C-section).

If you have low factor levels, here are other precautions you should take:

- Consult a hematologist before tooth extraction, surgery, or childbirth.
- Consider wearing a medical ID bracelet or necklace.
- Avoid products containing aspirin.
- Get a prescription for desmopressin

In other words, treat yourself like a person who has mild hemophilia. If you have any doubts, talk to your hematologist about what bleeds you might expect, and learn about proper treatment.

13 Deciding to Have More Children

PRENATAL TESTING

Once you've learned your carrier status and decided to become pregnant, you have more choices to make! You can let nature take its course, and give birth with no further genetic testing. Or you can have **prenatal testing** to determine two things:

- The sex of the fetus
- Whether a male fetus has hemophilia

Of course, you'll need to learn the sex of the fetus first. If you're having a girl, no more tests! If the baby is a boy, you can decide whether to have him tested prenatally for hemophilia. Some parents think that once they've learned it's a boy, they must test prenatally for hemophilia, but this isn't true. It's perfectly safe to give birth to your boy without having him tested in utero. Simply prepare for a safe birth as if your child has hemophilia, with all the necessary staff and tests ready.

Why would you choose to forgo testing? Some prenatal tests carry no risk; others carry a minimal risk of miscarriage.

Currently, there are four ways to prenatally check the sex of your baby:

- **Sonogram** (ultrasound)
- **Amniocentesis**
- **Chorionic villus sampling (CVS)**
- **Percutaneous blood sampling (PUBS)**

Sonogram

The easiest prenatal test to determine your baby's gender is a sonogram or ultrasound. A sonogram uses sound waves to take a picture of your unborn child, showing its gender, and poses no risk to the mother or child. Performed at 11 weeks of pregnancy and onward, an ultrasound's accuracy in determining gender increases with increased gestational age. At 11 weeks, it's about 70% accurate, at 12 weeks 92% accurate, and at 13 weeks greater than 98% accurate.[6] If you're having a girl, you can cancel further tests for hemophilia.

Amniocentesis

Amniocentesis is usually performed between weeks 15 and 16 of pregnancy. It involves inserting a long, thin needle through a pregnant woman's abdomen into the uterus, and removing a small sample of amniotic fluid from the amniotic sac around the fetus. The insertion of the needle and withdrawal of the fluid takes less than two minutes, and the whole process usually takes less than 30 minutes. In the fluid are cells shed from the fetus. These cells can be tested for a variety of birth defects. You can find out your baby's sex from nine days to two weeks after the test is performed. Some laboratories provide results in 24 hours. Amniocentesis has an accuracy rate greater than 99%. It carries a very small risk of miscarriage, but the amount of risk is often disputed.[7]

Chorionic villus sampling

CVS has an accuracy rate greater than 99%. The main advantage of this test over amniocentesis is that CVS can be performed earlier, between weeks 10 and 12 of pregnancy. CVS uses one of two techniques: (1) a long, thin needle is inserted through the abdomen into the placenta, or (2) a thin, flexible tube is inserted through the cervix. The needle or tube withdraws a sample of the chorionic villus, which are finger-like projections at the edge of the placenta. Similar to amniocentesis, the fetal cells drawn by CVS contain DNA and can be examined for genetic markers for hemophilia. Test results for your child's sex and for certain birth defects may be available in 48 hours. The test for hemophilia will take longer, and may not be available until after the first trimester, or around 12 weeks. About 1% of women tested with CVS (1 in 100) suffer a test-related miscarriage.

Percutaneous umbilical blood sampling

PUBS (also called cordocentesis) provides information about the risk of certain chromosomal blood disorders, including hemophilia. Performed after week 20, PUBS involves removing a sample of fetal blood from the umbilical vein. Results are normally available in a few days. PUBS is a highly specialized test that requires expertise to be performed safely, and may not be available at all hospitals. PUBS is slightly riskier than amniocentesis (the miscarriage rate is 1% to 3%) and is performed less often than amniocentesis. There are risks of side effects such as infection, cramping, and bleeding.

When you discuss prenatal testing with a genetics counselor, make sure you get specific information about the timing and accuracy of each type of test, the cost, and the relevance to your situation.

IT'S A BOY! NOW WHAT?

Some parents feel they have an emotional head start when they learn that their unborn child has hemophilia. They won't have the sudden shock of hearing their infant's diagnosis. Another major advantage is that they can make informed decisions about safe methods of delivery.

A vaginal birth should be a safe delivery method as long as forceps or vacuum extraction procedures are not used. But birth is naturally a traumatic process. Powerful uterine contractions compress the infant's head as it squeezes through the birth canal. In rare cases, this might be enough to cause an intracranial hemorrhage: a head bleed that occurs usually beneath the *dura mater*, the outer membrane that covers the spinal cord and brain.[8]

Fortunately, ICH is relatively uncommon, affecting fewer than 1 in 20 newborns with severe and moderate hemophilia. That's a fairly low 1% to 5% risk for these babies. But because the risk is so low, many physicians don't focus on ICH prevention. And poorly informed doctors may miss the signs of ICH and misdiagnose it, especially in children with no family history of hemophilia.

If you know you're a carrier, you'll want to prepare carefully for the birth of your baby boy. You'll either know that he *might* have hemophilia, or that he *does have* hemophilia because you've tested him. What steps should you take to ensure a safe delivery?

Before the birth:

1. Discuss birthing options with your obstetrician and a pediatric hematologist from the nearest HTC.

2. Make a plan for each step of the labor and delivery process.

3. Agree on delivery options in the event of unexpected complications. At what point during a vaginal birth would your obstetrician consider a C-section? If hospital staff suggest forceps or vacuum extraction, insist on a C-section.

4. If you're a carrier, have your baseline factor levels tested. Factor VIII levels will increase significantly during pregnancy, though factor IX levels do not change during pregnancy. Have your factor levels tested again during your third trimester, when levels are highest. Give the results to your obstetrician and anesthesiologist, and have them consult with your hematologist. If your levels are low, precautions should be taken during labor to prevent bleeding. Ask if you will you need a factor infusion before you deliver. Ask your obstetrician to insert written documentation of the team's conclusions into your file.

> **MASAC Recommendation 77**
>
> Adopted by NHF Board of Directors, February 22, 1998
> The majority of infants of hemophilia carriers can be safely delivered vaginally. Vacuum devices and instruments, such as internal fetal scalp monitors, should not be used because of the risk of bleeding.

During the birth:

1. Have your spouse or birth attendant act as your advocate during the delivery. You may be too focused on the birthing process to remind doctors that a long, difficult labor and the use of forceps and other devices to aid delivery can cause head bleeds in infants.[9]

2. If you're a carrier, give birth at a major hospital or HTC with staff experienced in hemophilia. Your child's birth and subsequent care is a team effort involving many medical and psychological specialists: genetics counselor, obstetrician, pediatrician, hematologist, nurses, HTC staff. Voice your opinion. Don't be afraid to replace medical staff if you don't trust them or they don't listen to you.

After the birth:

1. Avoid intramuscular injections, blood draws, and surgical procedures such as circumcision until the results of blood tests are known. Blood should be drawn from the umbilical cord (not your baby!) immediately after birth to check factor levels, confirm the diagnosis if needed, and perform other blood tests.[10]

2. Along with your pediatrician and nurses, monitor your baby closely during the first week. Where would he be best monitored: in your hospital room or the maternity nursery? If you had an epidural, talk to staff about differences in the symptoms of a post-epidural baby versus

a baby with a head bleed. Watch for signs of intracranial bleeding: listlessness, vomiting, poor feeding, unusual bruises. You may be tempted to trust the word of hospital staff that your infant is fine, even when he shows these symptoms. After all, these people deliver babies every day, right? But they don't deliver babies with hemophilia every day, so your advocacy is essential. Even if you need to rant to get cooperation, have your child tested for a head bleed if you think he shows symptoms.

3. Discuss whether postnatal tests are needed. Some experts advise a CT scan, MRI, or ultrasound within the first 24 hours for every newborn with severe or moderate hemophilia. Some recommend a factor infusion immediately following birth. Why? Because the symptoms of a head bleed aren't usually apparent for the first few days, and CT scans don't detect early head bleeds. While you're monitoring your child, an immediate infusion could stop a head bleed before damage is done. In one exceptional case, an infant was infused through the umbilical cord before he was born.

4. Document your delivery and follow-up care. Ask for copies of hospital records and physician orders. In the rare instance that your child has an undiagnosed bleed and medical staff reject your requests for factor therapy or scans, you'll have the evidence you need to support your case, in court if necessary.

5. Consult with your hematologist to prepare for the possibility of postpartum hemorrhaging. Factor VIII levels drop rapidly after childbirth, so if your factor levels are normally low, you may be at risk.

Remember that head bleeds following birth are rare. Most children with hemophilia arrive in the world safely—and loudly!

13 Deciding to Have More Children

A TRULY PERSONAL DECISION?

When you learn that you're a carrier, your decision to have more children is personal, but it will affect many. Look at practical matters, such as job security, health insurance coverage, and financial means. Can you continue at your current job when you have a child with a chronic disorder?

A child with severe hemophilia may eventually require several hundred thousand dollars' worth of factor every year. If he develops inhibitors, this may become millions of dollars every year, contributing to the rising cost of healthcare.

There are also psychosocial considerations: your ability to handle additional stress, your acceptance of responsibility for your child's medical care, and the kind of support you have from extended family. Should you bring another child into the world knowing he might have hemophilia?

Much depends on your individual circumstances, but even more depends on your beliefs about what's right for you and your responsibilities to society.

Some parents feel that one child with hemophilia is enough to handle. Other parents feel that biological siblings, with or without hemophilia, are worth the risk. Family planning decisions should involve both parents. You must consider opposing opinions, speak to your social worker, and examine your hearts, faith, and social responsibilities.

It's personal. It's your decision. A child with a chronic medical condition brings incalculable joy and growth, but also sober personal, family, and social responsibilities.

Understanding Your Insurance Coverage
Chapter 13 Summary

- Having more children is your decision, but you must accept responsibility for that decision. Know your probability of having a child with hemophilia.
- You are an obligate carrier if your father had hemophilia and you are female, you're the mother of more than one child with hemophilia, or you're a mother who has one child and another blood relative with hemophilia.
- If you're not sure whether you're a carrier, genetic tests can determine your carrier status.
- If you're a known carrier, your risk is 25% (1 in 4) of having a child with hemophilia.
- Prenatal testing can determine the sex of the fetus and whether a male fetus has hemophilia.
- You can determine sex by sonogram, amniocentesis, CVS, or PUBS. PUBS, CVS, and amniocentesis can also test for hemophilia in utero.
- Head bleeds caused by the birthing process are rare, but they do happen. Discuss birthing options with your obstetrician and a pediatric hematologist.
- Monitor your newborn closely during the first week, and watch for signs of cranial bleeding: listlessness, vomiting, poor feeding, or unusual bruises.

14

When an Inhibitor Strikes

We have said no to the town soccer league and to rollerblades—he'll tell you the jury is still out on that one—but he plays tennis, T-ball, and basketball. With the removal of his central line last year, he can finally swim. An inhibitor diagnosis can be scary, but it's not all doom and gloom. Leland is living a full life and having a ball! —Chris and Jane Smith, Massachusetts

By now you know that treating your child's bleeds means infusing factor concentrate to replace the missing factor in his bloodstream. But in some people with hemophilia, infusing standard factor doesn't work. The bleeding continues, despite the infusion. The person with hemophilia has developed an inhibitor.

Inhibitors are **antibodies**: blood proteins produced by the body's immune system. Antibodies are programmed to identify, cling to, and inactivate specific foreign invaders—such as viruses and bacteria—not recognized as a normal part of the body. Sometimes the body identifies infused factor as a foreign invader, creates an inhibitor, and inactivates the infused factor.

But why? Factor isn't a virus or bacteria. Why would the body neutralize factor? If either factor VIII or IX is not present in your child's fetal development, as is the often the case with severe hemophilia, his immune system may not recognize the missing factor as a normal component in his blood. Then, when factor is infused, his immune system is alerted. His body tries to neutralize the factor, just as it would a virus or bacteria. His immune system creates an inhibitor targeting the infused factor VIII or IX.[1]

When an inhibitor develops, hemophilia treatment with a standard factor concentrate may not work to stop a bleed. Scary? Yes, and this can be a grave complication of hemophilia, resulting in bleeds that last longer and produce more joint damage. Fortunately, today some inhibitors can be eliminated, and treatments exist that can control bleeds by bypassing the need for a specific clotting factor.

REACTING TO THE DIAGNOSIS

When you learn that your child has an inhibitor, you may revisit the cycle of grief and acceptance described in Chapter 1. Whether parents learn shortly after giving birth, or even when their child is a teenager, most experience a flood of emotion. One mother "swore like a sailor," and another felt "shock." One parent felt "betrayed," and another "furious." One mother described herself as "cheated."

"We went through the grief process yet again," recall Amy and Eric Walker. "Hearing the diagnosis of an inhibitor was like getting the diagnosis of hemophilia all over again, two years later." Still, the Walkers were glad to finally know why the factor had stopped working. They empowered themselves by looking for solutions and information to help manage their feelings. Knowledge can provide balance when you're thinking in drastic terms, like Nicole Olesen, who initially "thought it was a death sentence."

When you received the hemophilia diagnosis, your HTC staff was probably the single best place to get information. The same is true now: HTC staff can explain about the inhibitor and your treatment options. Treatment will vary depending on the type of inhibitor and the level of antibodies in your child's blood.

WHO'S LIKELY TO DEVELOP AN INHIBITOR?

Children may be born with hemophilia, but they are not born with an inhibitor to factor. Most people who develop an inhibitor also have severe factor deficiency, and this makes sense. Because they may have no factor, or factor that looks much different than it should, the immune system considers normal infused factor abnormal or dangerous, and targets it to be destroyed. Children with mild or moderate factor deficiency naturally have some factor active in the bloodstream, so the immune system is less likely to identify infused factor as a foreign material. That's why a child with mild or moderate hemophilia is much less likely to develop an inhibitor.

What chance does your child have of developing an inhibitor? Statistics on inhibitors can be confusing because various sources quote widely differing rates. Rates can vary between studies for many reasons: the size of the study sample (small samples common to many inhibitor studies can produce wide variation), the severity of hemophilia in the study population, the type of gene mutation causing the hemophilia, the length of the study, and so on.

To make sense of the stats, you need to know the difference between two types of measurements: **incidence** and **prevalence**.

> **Incidence:** the number of *new cases of inhibitors* in a given period of time. This includes inhibitors that spontaneously appear and then disappear.
>
> **Prevalence:** the number of cases of *long-standing inhibitors*. These are our focus in this chapter.

For inhibitors against factor VIII, the incidence is higher than the prevalence. This means that fewer people are living with inhibitors long term compared to the number who first develop inhibitors. Why? Because some inhibitors are transitory—they go away on their own—and others can be eliminated through treatment protocols.

For inhibitors against factor IX, the situation is reversed: the prevalence is higher than the incidence. This means that fewer inhibitors occur to begin with, but there are more people living with them long term because most of these inhibitors don't go away on their own, and they're harder to get rid of with treatment protocols.

Here's a clear way to understand the risk of developing an inhibitor:

- The incidence of inhibitors in people with severe factor VIII deficiency is 20% to 52%.
- The overall incidence of inhibitors in people with severe hemophilia is about 30%.
- The prevalence of inhibitors in people with severe factor VIII deficiency is 12% to 13%.
- The incidence of inhibitors in people with severe factor IX deficiency is 1% to 3%.
- The prevalence of inhibitors in people with severe factor IX deficiency is about 4%.[2]

For the best overall estimate of your child's risk, look at prevalence. And remember that not all inhibitors are alike. Some inhibitors are powerful, quickly inactivating all the infused factor. Some are weak, inactivating only some of the infused factor. And some children develop a transient inhibitor: it stays briefly, for weeks or months, and then disappears on its own.

Your child is more likely to develop an inhibitor if . . .

- he is factor VIII deficient,
- he has lower than 1% normal factor levels (severe),
- he is of African American or Hispanic heritage,
- he has a particular genetic defect predisposing him to an inhibitor,
- he has a relative with an inhibitor, or
- his first exposure to factor involves prolonged intensive factor therapy at a young age for surgery, after a major injury, or while ill.

Primary Risk Factor

The primary risk factor for developing an inhibitor is the type of gene mutation that causes the hemophilia. Although the overall incidence of inhibitors in hemophilia A is 30%, this varies depending on the type of mutation.

Gene mutations that do not produce a factor VIII protein are called "null."[3] These null mutations are associated with the highest rates of inhibitor formation. The single most common gene mutation resulting in severe hemophilia A is the intron 22 inversion. This null mutation accounts for almost one-half of all cases of severe hemophilia A; it happens when a section of the factor VIII gene is reversed, or inverted. The intron 22 mutation has an inhibitor incidence of 21%.

Two other types of null mutations can occur: (1) large deletions, where a big chunk of the gene is missing; and (2) nonsense mutations, when a mutated gene produces no factor. Together, these mutations have an inhibitor incidence of up to 88%. But luckily, they are relatively rare.[4]

Other Risk Factors

Does your choice of factor type or brand influence whether your child will develop an inhibitor? Though this question was debated for many years, the largest inhibitor study to date, the CANAL study, has determined that the type or brand of factor has little influence on whether your child will develop an inhibitor. There was also no evidence that switching factor products increased the inhibitor rate.[5]

Some parents think that giving their child "too much" factor can trigger an inhibitor. This is not true. Your child is *not* more likely to develop an inhibitor if he has frequent infusions. In fact, regular prophylaxis appears to have a protective effect and is associated with a 60% decrease in inhibitor risk!

But if your child's *first* exposure to factor happens during major surgery or a major bleed when he received factor for five or more consecutive days, then his risk of developing an inhibitor is three times higher than if he had received factor on a single day or two consecutive days. The risk is also more than three times higher if he receives high doses of factor (greater than 50 IU/kg) for five or more consecutive days, as compared to lower doses (less than 35 IU/kg). Consult with your hematologist to decide whether elective surgery, such as port implantation, can be delayed until after your child has been exposed to several factor infusions.

So don't limit or stop factor infusions in an attempt to prevent inhibitor development. The greatest risk of developing an inhibitor is associated with genetics, which you cannot control. Most inhibitors occur in young children when their immune systems are first being introduced or "challenged" with factor. According to the CANAL inhibitor study, half of all inhibitors occur before the 15th "exposure day" and the other half occur, with a sharply decreasing incidence rate, relatively soon afterward. By 50 exposure days, the risk of developing inhibitors decreases to less than 1%.

Research has shown that if a child hasn't developed an inhibitor by his 100th infusion, it's unlikely to happen. A child with severe hemophilia can reach his 100th infusion in one to three years with current therapy, or sooner with prophy. But in rare cases, teenagers and adults have developed inhibitors.

WHEN TO TEST FOR AN INHIBITOR?

How do you know if your child has an inhibitor? You may get a suspicion the hard way: factor infusions require higher doses and don't seem to be working, and your child's bleed continues or even worsens.

Fortunately, HTCs routinely test for an inhibitor. Testing is usually done at your child's annual comprehensive visit and before surgeries or invasive procedures. If your child has a surprisingly aggressive bleed or one that doesn't respond well to factor, you can request an inhibitor test (see next section).[6] Normally, circulating factor is slowly depleted at a rate according to its half-life. But if an inhibitor is present, factor is depleted at a rate faster than its normal half-life.

Inhibitor testing should *always* be done before surgery or other elective procedures such as tooth extractions or biopsies, even if your child has never tested positive for an inhibitor. Never take chances with surgery!

THE INHIBITOR TEST

The presence of an inhibitor is determined by a screening test called a Bethesda inhibitor assay, which measures the length of time it takes a mixture of the patient's plasma and normal plasma to form a clot.[7] A prolonged clotting time indicates an inhibitor.

The inhibitor level is measured in **Bethesda units** (BU) or **Bethesda titers**, reflecting the amount of inhibitor present. The inhibitor level is expressed as a number. The higher the number, the more antibodies in the blood, the more powerful the effect of the inhibitor, and the less effective a factor infusion will be.[8]

- A low-titer inhibitor is consistently less than 5 BU.
- A high-titer inhibitor is equal to or greater than 5 BU.[9]

Besides BU, an inhibitor is also classified according to how the immune system responds after being exposed to factor concentrate. If the inhibitor level remains stable or increases only slightly after being exposed to factor, but always remains below 5 BU, then it is a low-responding inhibitor. If it rises dramatically above 5 BU after factor exposure, called an **anamnestic response**, then it is classified as a high-responding inhibitor.

Low-responding inhibitor: infused factor will still work, but will have a significantly shorter half-life, so you must infuse higher factor doses to compensate for the factor inactivated by the inhibitor. Repeated factor infusions do not cause the inhibitor to rise above 5 BU.

High-responding inhibitor: infused factor may be completely inactivated, sometimes within minutes, and the bleed will continue.

Low-titer, low-responding inhibitors are fairly manageable, and bleeds can usually be treated with high doses of normal factor. Bleeds in the presence of high-titer, high-responding inhibitors can't usually be treated with normal factor concentrates and are harder to manage: special bypassing agents (see next section) are needed to treat bleeds.[10]

> **Good News About Inhibitors**
>
> - Most people with hemophilia do not get inhibitors.
> - People with hemophilia B, and those with moderate or mild hemophilia A, are much less likely than people with severe hemophilia to develop inhibitors.
> - Approximately 56% of hemophilia A patients who develop inhibitors develop low-titer, low-responding inhibitors. Of these inhibitors, about 39% are transient and will disappear on their own, typically within months. Another 26% of the low-responding inhibitors will resolve on their own over a period of several years.[11]

14 *When an Inhibitor Strikes*

TREATING INHIBITORS

Inhibitor risks, inhibitor levels, types of immune response . . . the possibilities can be confusing and frightening. But don't be overwhelmed: remember that some inhibitors are transient, disappearing with no intervention. Or they may be low-titer, low-responding inhibitors, so they don't have a major effect on normal factor therapy, and infused factor can still clot blood. Even when inhibitor levels are high and do affect normal factor therapy, you have several options. Some high inhibitors can be treated and even eradicated permanently!

There are two basic treatment options, which can be done separately or concurrently:

Treating bleeds
Eradicating the inhibitor

Option 1: Treating Bleeds

Bleeds can be treated directly with **bypassing agents** or with high doses of standard factor to overwhelm the inhibitor.

Bypassing agents. The following three types of factor concentrates are called bypassing agents because they skip the steps in the clotting process where factor VIII or IX is needed.

> **Prothrombin complex concentrates (PCCs):** plasma-derived factor concentrates that contain factors II, VII, IX, and X, and trace amounts of inactive factor VIII. They are usually unaffected by the factor VIII inhibitor because they don't require factor VIII or factor IX to form a clot. Remember that an inhibitor is created specifically to attack either factor VIII or IX and leaves the other clotting factors alone.

Activated prothrombin complex concentrates (aPCCs): PCCs that are "activated" during the manufacturing process. Activated means that some steps in the clotting process have already occurred, such as the function of factor VIII. The rest of the clotting process can continue without the need for factor VIII, so the immune system is not alerted when an aPCC is infused.

PCCs are often used for high-titer, high-responding inhibitors, which are hard to treat. They're also used for people with inhibitors and hemophilia B. As plasma-derived products, both PCCs and aPCCs can cause an anamnestic[12] response in people with hemophilia A because they contain trace amounts of inactive factor VIII. A small amount of factor VIII is sometimes all it takes to stimulate the immune system to boost an inhibitor.

Recombinant factor VIIa (rFVIIa; "a" stands for activated): products that, like PCCs and aPCCs, bypass the need for factor VIII. Activated factor VII, along with another protein called tissue factor, helps create a clot by activating factor X without the need for factor VIII or factor IX. This concentrate contains pure factor VII with no extraneous (unwanted) proteins and no other clotting factors, so the risk of anamnestic response for people with hemophilia A or hemophilia B is eliminated.

Porcine factor VIII (pig factor VIII): close enough to human factor VIII that it works in clotting human blood, but different enough to often escape detection by the immune system and not be inactivated by inhibitors to human factor VIII (though after exposure to porcine factor VIII, inhibitors may develop that inactivate it). Plasma-derived porcine factor VIII often causes allergic reactions and may cause a drop in blood platelets. It is not routinely used to treat bleeds in people with inhibitors, and in fact is no longer available on the market.

14 When an Inhibitor Strikes

High doses of standard factor. Frequent, high doses of standard factor concentrate are useful for people with low-titer inhibitors. The logic behind this is that the bloodstream becomes saturated with so much factor that the inhibitor can't possibly neutralize it all, and some will eventually work to clot the blood and stop a bleed.

Bypassing products can effectively control bleeds even with high-titer inhibitors. One major medical concern is that they can clot blood so successfully that some patients risk thrombosis. Thrombosis is the formation of blood clots, which can prevent blood from flowing normally through a blood vessel, possibly causing a stroke. Thrombosis can result if your child with an inhibitor is dosed too often, overdosed, or treated after receiving a crush injury. You and your HTC team should discuss thrombosis when choosing an inhibitor treatment protocol.

Inhibitor levels may also be temporarily reduced (for example before surgery) to allow standard factor concentrates to be used, with one of these processes:

Plasmapheresis: the patient's blood is passed slowly through a machine that removes the plasma and replaces it with fresh plasma or a substitute. Replacing 3 or 4 liters of plasma in an adult can reduce an inhibitor level by 40% or more. Plasmapheresis can be used to lower the inhibitor level before elective surgery, and also to lower the inhibitor temporarily to prepare for ITT (see next section). Plasmapheresis takes several hours and is not routinely used to treat bleeds.

Immunoadsorption: during plasmapheresis, the removed plasma is passed through a device that physically removes the inhibitor from the plasma. This process is more efficient at removing inhibitors than plasmapheresis alone.

Option 2: Eradicating the Inhibitor

Most of the inhibitor treatments we've discussed so far are used to stop individual bleeds. But one treatment attempts to eradicate the inhibitor itself. **Immune tolerance therapy** desensitizes the body to factor VIII or factor IX permanently, so it stops producing an inhibitor when factor is infused. During ITT, daily high-dose factor infusions bombard your child's bloodstream with so much factor that eventually, his body tires of trying to neutralize it all and may stop producing an inhibitor. Through ITT, his body can "learn" to recognize factor in the bloodstream.

Make the decision about trying ITT soon after your child's inhibitor diagnosis. The success rate of ITT is higher for people who develop an inhibitor before age 5 and lower for those who develop an inhibitor after age 10. The success rate of ITT is higher if the inhibitor level has never been above 10 BU. And low-responding inhibitors are more easily eradiated than high-responding inhibitors. Young patients, including infants and toddlers, usually need a port to make it easier to give treatments. You'll be infusing a lot of factor, and you'll want to spare those little veins some wear and tear.

The protocol for ITT differs with each child. Typically, children receive up to 100 IU of factor per kilogram of body weight daily. Some receive less, some more. Some children need ITT for a few weeks, some for a few months, and some for a year or more. Doctors often tell families to be prepared to stay on ITT for up to three years. Even if the inhibitor is successfully eradicated, your hematologist may suggest prophy two to three times a week, regardless of whether your child has a bleed, to help his body continue to recognize factor in the bloodstream.

How good is ITT at treating inhibitors? In 70% to 80% of cases, ITT has successfully desensitized the immune system to factor VIII, resulting in very low inhibitor titers or complete elimination of the inhibitor. Therapy is considered successful if the inhibitor drops low enough that factor VIII can again be used effectively to treat bleeds. The success rate in eliminating factor IX inhibitors with ITT is much lower, only 31%.[13]

The success of ITT can't be guaranteed. And there are several different ITT treatment protocols. Even doctors and researchers haven't determined the optimal ITT protocol.

But one thing is certain: ITT requires commitment and teamwork from the family and HTC staff. The family needs to comply with guidelines established by the HTC—infusing the correct amount daily, keeping detailed records, and alerting staff to problems, such as breakthrough bleeds or port infections. HTC staff needs to determine if the family is capable of handling this responsibility, and if the child can tolerate it emotionally. Staff must prepare families adequately for this enormous commitment, by teaching them to implement the ITT program and guiding them through each stage of therapy.

INHIBITORS AND QUALITY OF LIFE

When you spend time with families who live with inhibitors, you may feel like you're talking about two different disorders. Lifestyles may differ drastically. Concerns may differ, too. The family without inhibitors may worry about whether their child can play soccer or when to remove a port; the family with inhibitors may worry about losing insurance, finding a product that works, managing pain, and preventing joint damage. Ziva Mann, mother of a child with an inhibitor, says, "It was frightening, and any bleeds would just take over my day. I'd drop everything and start doing a series of infusions."

If your child has an inhibitor, how will your daily life be affected? It's hard to say. Each child's experience is unique. If your child doesn't respond well to inhibitor treatment, should you prevent him from being active? Should you try to protect him from all injuries?

Some children can continue leading fairly normal lives in spite of inhibitors, attending school and being physically active. But because inhibitors prolong bleeds, this can mean pain, missed school, inactivity, or social isolation. Your child may feel angry, sad, or confused. *You* may feel angry, sad, or confused! Your biggest problem may be the tendency to be overprotective while you're waiting to find an effective therapy.

You can't prevent an inhibitor from forming, and sometimes you can't find an effective treatment. What you *can* do is learn to live with the inhibitor. Overcome your sense of helplessness by educating yourself and becoming active in your child's treatment. There are national programs that invite parents to meet, talk, and learn about inhibitors. Ask your hematologist lots of questions, and investigate various treatment options with your HTC. Request literature from HANDI at NHF. Order *Managing Your Child's Inhibitor*, an in-depth guidebook to living with inhibitors (see Appendix A). Treat inhibitors the way you've learned to handle all things hemophilia: be proactive, ask questions, read, and don't give up.

Fortunately, research is underway to determine exactly which parts of the factor protein elicit an immune response, and why some people develop inhibitors but others don't. Eventually we may be able to reduce the formation of inhibitors by modifying the factor protein so it doesn't trigger an immune response. New recombinant products, created from human cell lines instead of mammalian cell lines, are being developed in the hope of reducing the chance of inhibitor formation. Inhibitors are still a feared and challenging complication of hemophilia, yet the outlook and community support for people with inhibitors has never been brighter or stronger.

When an Inhibitor Strikes
Chapter 14 Summary

- An inhibitor is an antibody created by the body's immune system to inactivate factor VIII or factor IX, preventing infused factor from clotting blood.
- The prevalence of inhibitors in people with severe factor VIII deficiency is 12% to 13%, and up to 4% in people with severe factor IX deficiency.
- More than half of all inhibitors are either transient or low responding.
- An inhibitor titer is measured in Bethesda units (BU).
- An inhibitor may be low titer, low responding (less than 5 BU); or high titer, high responding (5 BU to over 1,000 BU), depending on how much it rises in reaction to infused factor.
- A child is more likely to develop an inhibitor if he has severe factor VIII deficiency, is of African American or Hispanic heritage, has a genetic predisposition to develop inhibitors, or has a relative with an inhibitor, or if his first exposure to factor involved prolonged intensive factor therapy at a young age for surgery, after a major injury, or while ill.
- Treatment to control bleeding with an inhibitor includes PCCs and aPCCs; recombinant factor VIIa; or, for low-responding inhibitors, high doses of factor to overwhelm the inhibitor.
- ITT is a treatment protocol designed to eradicate an inhibitor. ITT requires high doses of factor, usually daily, to desensitize the body to factor VIII or factor IX.
- ITT is successful in eliminating up to 80% of factor VIII inhibitors and up to 30% of factor IX inhibitors.
- Your HTC is the first stop for inhibitor information and treatment.

∽ 15 ∽

Understanding Your Insurance Coverage

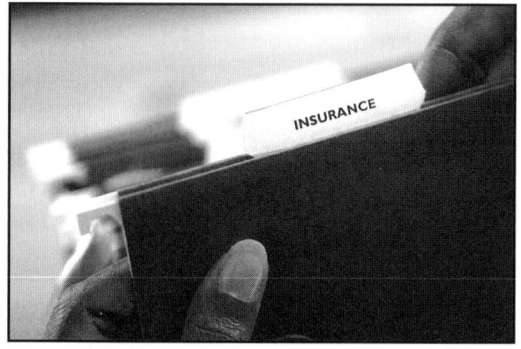

Deal seriously with insurance companies. Keep notes and lists, and prepare questions ahead of time. Don't take initial reactions (including ignorance) personally—the customer service reps are struggling with an unpredictable system. Get things in writing. Keep calling until your questions are answered. Try not to get emotional. I wasn't able to handle insurance problems when my son was first diagnosed. I had too much anger, fear, and emotion tied up with the process. But I've learned to move through it. It gets easier. If all else fails, eat ice cream! — Rita Epstein, New York

We're fortunate to live in the country that produces most of the world's factor, and some of the world's highest-quality factor. Factor in the United States is both safe and abundant. But factor is also one of the most expensive medicines. It's essential that you have some form of health insurance to pay for your factor concentrate and healthcare services—indeed, it's mandatory by law. You'll need to learn how to obtain insurance, make sure it covers the hemophilia care you need, and protect it from changes that threaten to limit hemophilia care.

Healthcare insurance continues to undergo massive reform in America. The **Affordable Care Act** (ACA) of 2010 changed many aspects of healthcare. Lifetime caps and preexisting condition exclusions are gone, but the ACA's individual mandate requires you and your dependents to have health insurance from at least one of these sources:

- a government-sponsored plan (Medicare, Medicaid),
- an employer-sponsored plan,
- a plan purchased through the Health Insurance Marketplace,
- grandfathered plans, or
- a state health benefits risk pool plan.

No matter which type of plan you choose or must accept, to preserve access to the medication you need and to your preferred providers, you must learn all you can about your personal insurance policy.[1] You'll need to know the answers to these questions:

- Who pays for my hemophilia care?
- How could insurance reforms affect my choices?
- Which kind of policy do I have?
- What does my policy cover, and what doesn't it cover?
- How will I manage costs?
- How will I maintain my health insurance coverage (see Chapter 16)?

WHO PAYS FOR INSURANCE?

In Chapter 6, we identified the various players in the hemophilia marketplace. These include insurance carriers—payers—because they reimburse the factor and healthcare services we use.

In the United States, health insurance is mostly commercial.[2] Private employers buy health insurance for their employees from private insurance companies such as Blue Cross Blue Shield Association, Cigna, and Aetna. Policies are also sold to individuals. Private insurance, through group and individual policies, covers about half of Americans with hemophilia.

15 *Understanding Your Insurance Coverage*

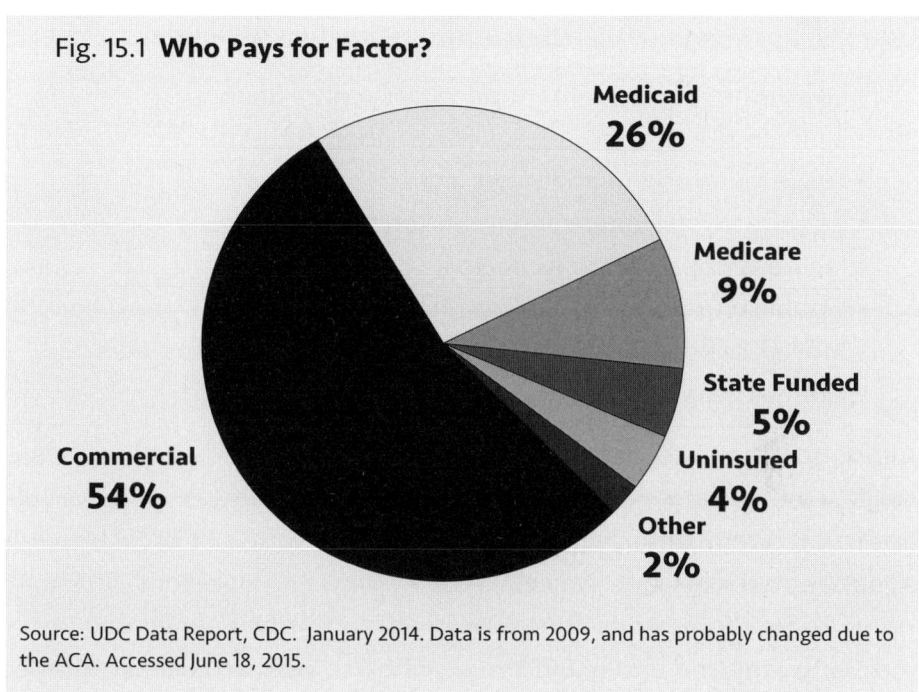

Fig. 15.1 **Who Pays for Factor?**

Medicaid **26%**
Medicare **9%**
State Funded **5%**
Uninsured **4%**
Other **2%**
Commercial **54%**

Source: UDC Data Report, CDC. January 2014. Data is from 2009, and has probably changed due to the ACA. Accessed June 18, 2015.

Public programs also exist to help people with their healthcare coverage. Medicaid helps low-income people, and **Medicare** is for people aged 65 and older, as well as people with certain chronic conditions. Of Americans with hemophilia, as of this writing, about 26% use Medicaid and 9% use Medicaid.[3]

Are you covered by private insurance or by a state or federally funded program? That's the first thing you need to know in order to manage your health insurance.

HEMOPHILIA HIGH ON INSURANCE RADAR

Recall from Chapter 6 that payers are becoming more prominent and powerful in the hemophilia marketplace, as they scrutinize all healthcare costs—particularly high-cost treatments—and seek ways to cut costs.

How will payers cut costs? Here are some of their methods:

- Lower the reimbursement price per unit of factor.
- Limit choice of factor brand or provider.
- Move factor to the pharmacy benefit side.
- Require prior authorization of all factor shipments.
- Increase copayments for factor.
- Establish preferred drug lists (PDLs).
- Move biologic products, like factor, to specialty drug tiers.
- Contract with pharmacy benefit managers (PBMs).[4]

Although everyone acknowledges the need to reduce healthcare costs, cost cutting could interfere with the quality of your child's treatment. Why? Unfortunately, payers sometimes don't know enough about hemophilia when they make budget-cutting decisions. So it may be up to you to educate them! You can do this best when you know their language and understand your policy, so you can challenge payer policy changes that might cut essential services and the therapy you need.

WHICH KIND OF INSURANCE DO YOU HAVE?

Once you've determined whether you have private or public insurance, you need to know the type of insurance plan you have under your policy: traditional or nontraditional. Most insurance plans can be classified as traditional *indemnity* plans or nontraditional *managed care* plans.

Traditional Indemnity Plans

About 10% of hemophilia patients with private insurance use traditional indemnity plans, also called Fee-for-Service (FFS). These plans generally allow more choice than nontraditional plans. With a traditional FFS plan,

- You can choose your own doctor.
- You don't need a referral from your primary care physician (PCP) to see a specialist.
- You may have a deductible (annual amount you must pay before your plan begins to pay).
- You may have a copay (amount you must pay per doctor visit, procedure, or prescription).
- You may need to fill out claim forms for each visit.
- You may have an annual maximum for nonessential health benefits (limit or **cap** on the amount of money paid for your nonessential health benefits medical expenses each year).

Expenses differ with various FFS plans. To estimate your annual out-of-pocket expenses per year, you need to ask about each portion of your policy. For example, you will pay a portion of your medical costs out-of-pocket (the deductible, typically 20%), up to a certain maximum per year, before the plan starts paying 100% of the allowable charge. The allowable charge is the amount the insurance company allows for a doctor visit or procedure, and is usually based on a community standard. Your annual deductible could be as low as $100 or as high as $1,500. This could be per person or per family.

You may have a lot of paperwork with FFS plans. Usually, you must fill in a claim form for each medical treatment or doctor's visit, pay for the visit or treatment, and then be reimbursed by the insurance company. It's vital to keep accurate records.

Nontraditional Managed Care Plans

Most American employees use some kind of nontraditional plan, also called a managed care plan, through a managed care organization (MCO). In general, MCOs attempt to contain rising healthcare costs by managing your use of medical services, by allowing less freedom of choice than FFS plans. For example, they may require you to use doctors, hospitals, or pharmacies approved by the insurance company as part of its network. MCOs are used by both private and public insurers.

In MCOs, the PCP is often called the gatekeeper. The PCP controls access to specialists (such as hematologists) and decides which diagnostic tests are necessary. Some MCOs pay PCPs a flat amount per patient per month to manage the healthcare needs of a group of patients—a process called *capitation*. Here's how it works: The group of patients to be managed can range from a few hundred to a few thousand people. If a patient needs to see a specialist, the cost of the specialist visit is deducted from the amount of money the PCP receives every month to treat that particular patient. Critics of capitation say that this payment system allows money to affect the doctor-patient relationship, creating an ethical dilemma for doctors. But you need specialists, because many PCPs have limited knowledge of hemophilia. Make sure your PCP is a team player willing to work with the HTC. Your child must be treated by a hematologist.

If you have a managed care plan, you will have one of three basic types:

Health Maintenance Organization (HMO). The healthcare provider also is the payer in this prepaid plan. You or your employer pay a monthly or quarterly fee, which often insures you for 80% to 100% of all medical costs, including hospitalization. You also may be charged an additional amount, or copay, for certain services such as office visits, outpatient surgery, and prescriptions. You are required to use HMO network doctors, who can refer you to in-network specialists, such as a pediatric hematologist. If your PCP's knowledge of hemophilia is limited, you may need to assert yourself to get to a hemophilia specialist. You must use HMO-approved hospitals, which may or may not include your HTC. Advantages? You shouldn't have to process any bills because they are sent to the HMO, and out-of-pocket costs are low. Drawbacks? Your choice of medical services is limited. And if you need to go out-of-network, expect to pay a higher price.

Preferred Provider Organization (PPO) or Exclusive Provider Organization (EPO). These plans offer more choice, better out-of-network benefits, and fewer restrictions than HMOs. They also offer reduced copays and lower deductibles when you use in-network doctors and hospitals. Going out-of-network is allowed but may mean higher copays. An EPO may not cover services outside its plan. Both PPO and EPO plans usually require prior authorization for hospitalization, for most outpatient procedures, and for expensive medicines like factor concentrate.

Point-of-Service (POS). One of the most rapidly expanding forms of managed care in the marketplace today, the POS plan offers flexible options. Consumers can use in-network healthcare providers at a reduced cost (HMO option) or out-of-network providers (traditional indemnity options). But increased freedom to choose out-of-network providers means higher monthly premiums and copays. Some employers simply add a POS plan to an already existing managed care plan, and employees can choose the existing plan or the POS plan. Some employers allow employees to sign up for the POS option and pay extra only if the POS plan is actually used. This is called a dual option program because the employee always has two options.

WHICH SERVICES ARE COVERED BY YOUR PLAN?

Whether you have a traditional or nontraditional plan, you need to know exactly which services and products are covered, or budgeted, under your current policy. The insurance company is required by law to provide you with an easy-to-understand summary of your benefits and coverage in writing in a "summary of benefits" document. *Never assume that coverage exists for any aspect of hemophilia.* To ensure that your plan covers the necessary providers and medications for your child, you'll need to *read your entire policy.* Be sure to ask questions if you're unsure about what specific benefits are included in your coverage.

All health insurance plans are required by the ACA to cover 10 essential health benefits:

- Ambulatory patient services
- Emergency services
- Hospitalization
- Maternity and newborn care
- Mental health and substance use disorder services, including behavioral health treatment
- Prescription drugs
- Rehabilitative and habilitative services and devices
- Laboratory services
- Preventive and wellness services and chronic disease management
- Pediatric services, including oral and vision care

These are broad categories, so you'll need to review your policy carefully to make sure that coverage exists for all aspects of hemophilia care.

A health insurance plan has two parts, representing two different budgets:

Medical benefit: (also called major medical) covers all clinical services, such as doctor visits, diagnostic tests, and surgery
Pharmacy benefit: covers outpatient drugs

For most people with hemophilia, factor is covered under the medical benefit. To cut costs, some insurance companies are moving factor to the pharmacy benefit. This shifts more costs onto patients. How? By requiring an out-of-pocket payment based on percentage of factor costs. So when factor is covered under the pharmacy benefit, be aware of copays! These out-of-pocket maximums, typically $3,000 to $5,000 annually, must be paid before prescription drugs are covered at 100%. Some plans have higher out-of-pocket maximums and cost-sharing requirements of up to 50% of the cost of factor. Out-of-pocket limits set by the ACA put a ceiling on your costs, but the out-of-pocket limit

15 Understanding Your Insurance Coverage

under the law exceeds $6,600 for an individual and $13,200 for a family, with limits rising every year.

Be sure that your factor brand is covered! Your plan may use a drug formulary. A formulary is a list of prescription drugs that are approved and covered by an insurance plan for its members. If your factor brand is not in the formulary, it may not be covered. Before you enroll in any plan, find out if the plan uses a formulary, and if your factor brand and all necessary medicines and supplies are on it.

Regardless of which plan you use, you need to know what's covered under your current policy and how—through the medical or pharmacy benefit. Ask these questions to find out what your plan covers:

1. When is open enrollment? Open enrollment, usually a 30-day period, is the one time annually when you have the opportunity to change health plans, even if you have Medicare. It's essential to know when open enrollment will occur, in case you need to find a better plan.

2. Is factor covered? If factor isn't considered a drug, it may be covered under the patient's medical benefit side of the policy.

3. Is there a copay for prescriptions? This can get expensive when you're ordering factor. Copays will count toward your annual out-of-pocket limit and your deductible.

4. Are there brand restrictions? Does the plan have a formulary or a PDL?[5] Is your brand of factor covered?

5. How is factor delivered? By hospital outpatient pharmacy, 340B program, specialty pharmacy, home care company, or mail-order company? Do you have choice of provider? Does your payer try to influence you to use its preferred provider?

6. Does the plan allow you to see your preferred healthcare provider?[7] Can you receive care at your HTC and from your preferred hematologist?

7. What costs are associated with the plan? These include deductible, copay, and coinsurance costs, all of which add up and count toward your annual out-of-pocket limit.

8. What is the monthly premium for the plan? When you're choosing a plan, you'll need to consider whether you want to pay a higher monthly premium or lower annual deductible. This budget preference must be factored into your decision.

9. Is there an annual maximum for services? For example, your insurer may put a cap on the number of physical therapy sessions a patient can have in a year.

10. Is prophylactic treatment covered? In contrast to on-demand therapy, prophylaxis can dramatically increase the cost of hemophilia medical care in the short term.

11. Is home treatment covered? Treating your child at home can significantly reduce medical costs. Will your plan allow you to home infuse? Store factor concentrate at home? Use a home care company to deliver factor? Hire a home infusion nurse?

12. Does the policy have riders? Riders are legal documents that modify or amend coverage under an insurance policy. For example, riders may be linked to dental and eyewear coverage. How will riders affect your benefits?

13. Is prior authorization needed to see a specialist, run tests, or receive other services? Along with the possibility of needing prior authorization to receive a certain brand of factor or prophy, prior authorization may be required for a variety of healthcare services. Check your policy carefully.

Fortunately, your child won't need to worry about tackling all of these health insurance questions for a while. Parents with a health insurance plan that already covers children can add or keep their children on the policy until age 26. This part of the ACA applies even if the child is married, is not living with you, is attending school, is not financially dependent on you, or is eligible to enroll in an employer's plan.

Mind-boggling, isn't it? The American insurance system is complicated, and you need to learn about it to protect your child's well-being. At the very least, remember this: *Never accept a health insurance policy without first knowing the answers to these questions—in writing.*

MANAGING COSTS

Even when you have a great insurance policy, understand your coverage, and have answers in writing, you still need to contain premium and out-of-pocket costs. Once a year, during open enrollment, you have the opportunity to keep your current health plan or enroll in another. This is when you'll need to determine if a premium increase or other change will occur in any of the coverage in your current plan. Then you can decide whether to choose a different plan that meets all your needs and keeps your costs down.

For out-of-pocket costs, the ACA sets a limit. This amount increases annually with the rate of premium adjustment percentage—the percentage by which the average per-person premium for health insurance coverage for the current calendar year exceeds the average per-person premium for the previous year. It's possible for the annual out-of-pocket limit to stay the same from one year to the next, but don't count on this. Your insurer might also set an out-of-pocket maximum for your plan that is lower than the one set by the ACA. Check with your human resources department or insurance provider to find out what the limit is each year.

Costs that can count toward the maximum out-of-pocket costs include deductibles, copays, and coinsurance. Monthly premiums never count toward your out-of-pocket maximum. But beware! Not all health insurance plans count your deductible, for example, toward your out-of-pocket maximum. Health insurers continue to find ways to put a greater burden of healthcare costs on the patient. Know what counts toward your out-of-pocket maximum in your plan.

The greatest cost in hemophilia treatment is the cost of factor. As insurers move factor to the pharmacy benefit side of your policy, an insurer may put factor on a *specialty tier* in its drug formulary. Tiers separate drugs into classifications, and determine how much of a drug's cost a patient will be required to pay. The traditional three-tier drug formulary used by most plans includes generics (tier 1); preferred brand-name drugs (tier 2); and non-preferred brand-name drugs (tier 3). Many plans now have added a specialty tier. Specialty tiers are for biologics, like factor, that are expensive to produce.

Insurers are using specialty tiers as a way to shift more of the cost of factor onto the patient. The out-of-pocket cost of a specialty tier drug can be high. Insurers can charge a percentage of the drug's cost, ranging from 20% to 33% and higher, rather than a fixed copay, like $10 per prescription refill for generic drugs. Imagine paying 33% of your factor costs every month!

It's best to prepare an annual budget for costs associated with treating your child's hemophilia. Before you can estimate your costs and assess when during the year you might reach your out-of-pocket maximum, you'll need to find out what your copay or coinsurance costs will be for factor, and what other medical costs you may incur. For the following costs, determine the exact amounts based on what's in your current insurance policy, or make an estimate based on past policies:

- Annual policy premium (for a group plan, multiply the amount taken out of each paycheck by the number of paychecks you receive yearly)
- Copay amount or coinsurance percentage for tests or any medical procedure (this will be an estimate)
- Annual deductible per person
- Annual out-of-pocket maximum per family as set by your plan and what counts toward that maximum
- Annual prescription costs for all medication, including factor (this will be an estimate)

Some costs are unpredictable: emergency surgery, hospitalization, and unscheduled doctor's visits. Other costs are predictable: HTC visits, prophy, and even factor costs related to specific bleeding patterns. Try to calculate predictable costs. You may choose to include in your estimate some amount for emergencies and unscheduled doctor's visits.

Now that you have an estimate of your annual expenses, you can break down this cost estimate into (1) an estimate of your healthcare costs for care and testing, and (2) an estimate of your factor costs. The following suggestions will help you manage these costs:

Plan for reaching your out-of-pocket maximum. Based on your estimate for your annual out-of-pocket costs, determine how much you will spend on health insurance, healthcare, and medication per month. Add an estimate of what you'd need for an emergency. Be aware of when you might reach your out-of-pocket maximum; such costs can be incurred quickly, possibly within first few months of the year.

Work with healthcare providers to help ensure that all services fall under essential health benefits as defined by the ACA. Ask in advance why a procedure is being ordered, how much it costs, and whether it's covered by your health insurance. Is the procedure medically necessary? Is it being ordered to legally cover the medical team?

Investigate the patient assistance programs offered by many home care and pharmaceutical companies.[6] These companies can work with you to contain costs. If you can prove financial hardship, they may waive certain fees or portions of the bill (see Chapter 16).

Explore home infusion. Home infusion saves money. Avoid the ER unless you have a true emergency, your HTC or urgent care center is closed, or your HTC is far from home. Check with your HTC about alternate, local options for urgent medical assistance.

Get an HSA (pretax health savings account). Estimate costs, and put money toward the HSA. Funds in your HSA cover qualified medical expenses as described in Section 213(d) of the Internal Revenue Service Tax Code. You can set aside an annual maximum every year in an HSA. This amount changes annually, so check with your human resources department or HealthCare.gov for each year's maximum. For a list of qualified medical expenses, visit the IRS website.

Consider a secondary insurance plan. You can obtain one through your employer or on your own. You can usually submit your copays for coverage and reimbursement through the secondary plan, which will lower your costs. But explore this option only if the premiums will be less overall than your anticipated costs when using a single plan.

Coordinate benefits through insurance plans when possible. If you and your spouse already have separate insurance policies, you may be able to increase your coverage by coordinating benefits through both plans.

RECORD, DOCUMENT, FILE

Every visit to the doctor or hospital, every lab test, every service, and every factor order generates medical expenses and medical bills. Eventually, the medical service provider or factor provider will invoice your payer, who will provide the reimbursement. Your payer may send you a copy of the explanation of benefits (**EOB**). This is a document sent to patients by the insurance company that lists medical services received and reimbursed. You should receive an EOB after every medical service. The medical provider will bill you if you owe a copay or coinsurance payment, or bill for any product or service not covered by your insurance policy.

From day one, you must keep comprehensive, accurate records of all your EOBs, your insurance policy, and any other relevant records. To track your expenses and services, now is the time to set up a filing system, perhaps in a portable file case or on your computer. You never know when you'll need your records as evidence of coverage and payment, to phone your payer or even to present in court.

The time may come when you and your payer will disagree about costs, payments, and coverage. Always keep accurate records of

- all medical procedures,
- any phone calls with your payer, and
- all written correspondence with your payer.

Medical procedures include infusions, hospital trips, services received, tests, and doctor visits. Keep records of everything for at least three years to help you determine whether your deductible has been met; assess your portion of costs; decide if you're being billed fairly; and see how, if, and when during each procedure you are reaching your out-of-pocket maximum. Consider setting up a chart to track each illness and injury.

Records are essential when you have many bleeds, are covered by two insurance policies, or pay a portion of the bills. Healthcare providers and insurance companies do make errors in billing: for example, charging for nonexistent services, billing twice, or overbilling. Protect your own finances by tracking errors. Carefully read and file the EOB.

Always photocopy or scan your claim forms and any correspondence with the hospital or insurance company. You can question and petition errors from a position of strength if you have detailed records to back up your claim.

Take notes on phone conversations with your insurance company representatives. Someday you may need to know exactly who spoke with you and what was said. Document full names, titles, time and date of call, subject, and conclusion. Ask for direct phone numbers instead of extensions. You may be assigned a case number when you call. Ask for and record all case numbers.

If you call to ask about alternate insurance policies, *you do not have to identify yourself*. You can ask about hemophilia without revealing your name, address, or Social Security number. If questioned, politely explain that you don't wish to be identified. Once you've received satisfactory answers from the insurance company, follow up: get all those answers in writing. *Document everything, and get everything documented!*

CLAIM DENIED? HOW TO APPEAL

If payment is denied for a service or medicine you need, you can appeal the denial and challenge the insurance company's decision.[7] All insurance companies have an appeals procedure. Here are some things to remember when appealing a decision:

The squeaky wheel gets the grease. If you think your claim has been unfairly denied, pursue it without hesitation. Claims are repeatedly denied in the hope that the person will stop pursuing payment. Report your suspicions to the insurance commissioner in your state.

Educate the insurance company. Give the claims examiner some information about hemophilia. Ask your doctor or HTC to supply documentation to support your case.

Know what your policy offers. This helps you determine whether your insurance company has denied a covered benefit appropriately.

Get the reason for the denial in writing. This document should contain the reason for the denial and the name and title of the person who reviewed your claim. By law, your insurer must provide this to you.

Get a written copy of your insurance company's appeal process. The ACA requires your insurance company to provide it. Follow this process as you make your appeal. The timeline for the standard appeals process may be too long if it's more than a few days, and if it might put your life at risk or affect your ability to function normally, preventing you from working or caring for yourself and others. In this case, you can file an appeal for an expedited decision. If you meet the standards for an expedited external review, the final decision about your appeal must come as quickly as your medical condition requires, and no later than 72 hours after your request for external review is received.

Write a formal letter to appeal the denial. Include all the facts of your case that support your need for the treatment or procedure. If the benefit you're seeking should be covered according to your policy, then state in your letter that you expect the insurer to fulfill its contractual obligations. Use the letter template in Appendix C.

Include hemophilia standard-of-care or treatment guidelines. Find a copy of standards of care in NHF's MASAC recommendations (www.hemophilia.org).

Consider a second medical opinion. To strengthen your appeal, you may want to submit to the insurance company a second medical opinion from a doctor specializing in hemophilia.

Leave a paper trail. Keep copies of all written correspondence with your insurance company. Send all your correspondence Certified Mail with Return Receipt requested, so you have proof that your mail was received.

Maintain records of conversations with your insurance company. Note dates, times, and names of insurance company representatives. Remember that weeks, even months, will pass during the appeal.

Enlist reimbursement experts from your HTC, home care company, and pharmaceutical manufacturer. Ask your local hemophilia foundation and state insurance commissioner for help.

If the internal appeal is denied, ask for a third-party appeal. Under the ACA, all insurance companies are required to allow you to have an external third party review your appeal.

If all else fails, consider legal recourse. Do any legal clinics in your community assist with claims denials on a free or low-cost basis? Your state bar association may be able to help.

Simply understanding your basic health insurance policy is daunting. Appealing a claim forces you even deeper into the insurance maze. You'll need help navigating this maze, and help is available from many sources. You'll never have to go it alone!

HEMOPHILIA WITH BENEFITS

Of all the things you must learn about hemophilia, insurance may be the most complex and frustrating, but certainly the most needed. Insurance is a rapidly changing field. Keep abreast of changes by reading NHF and HFA publications, *PEN*, and publications from pharmaceutical companies and home care companies. Talk to your HTC social worker, employer, and state insurance commissioner's office.

People are waiting to help you, but they can help only if you do your part. Know your insurance coverage, keep accurate records, update your child's personal medical information annually, and question everything. Health insurance is a necessity for people with hemophilia. Never take it for granted. Never be complacent or assume that someone else will take care of it. Only you can know your plan and your needs. Only *you* can monitor changes and prepare for the future of healthcare. Insurance is tough, but parents of children with hemophilia are tougher—a rare breed, and you are one of them!

Understanding Your Insurance Coverage
Chapter 15 Summary

- Hemophilia is one of the most expensive of all chronic disorders.
- Insurance payers provide financial coverage for hemophilia expenses. Payers include private insurance companies and public programs, such as Medicaid and Medicare.
- The ACA of 2010 created many benefits for families with hemophilia, including no annual and lifetime caps, no preexisting condition exclusions, and a longer time that adult children can stay on their parents' plans.
- Understand your insurance policy: Is factor covered? How is it delivered? Is prophylactic treatment covered? Is home treatment covered? Are there riders?
- Estimate your annual out-of-pocket costs and the time during the year when you will incur these costs. Plan accordingly. Ask your HTC social worker to help you estimate your annual costs. Download a copy of NHF's Insurance Toolkit to assist you.
- Keep accurate records of all medical procedures, EOBs, claims, and any phone calls and correspondence with your insurance company.
- Insurance is a rapidly changing field. Keep abreast of changes by reading current publications and asking questions.

16

Maintaining Your Insurance Coverage

I have insurance through my employer. There's a high deductible. We meet our deductible and out-of-pocket with the first order of factor, which I try to time at the beginning of our insurance year. I qualify for financial aid with our home care company, so the out-of-pocket is covered: all our medical expenses and prescriptions are paid for 100% for the rest of the year. That's one positive in all the setbacks and heartaches of having a child with hemophilia. —Mary Boudreaux, Texas

Before the Affordable Care Act, one of the most frightening scenarios for a family with hemophilia was losing health insurance. Families and individuals could lose their health insurance when they changed jobs, resigned, or were laid off; when they reached a lifetime cap in health benefits; or if their employer cancelled their insurance.

Now that the ACA is in effect, what has changed? What can you do if you're threatened with losing your health insurance?

First, don't panic. Because the ACA requires all US citizens and their dependents to have health insurance, the act provides two options to maintain health insurance coverage. You can

- sign up for a Health Insurance Marketplace plan, or
- go on **COBRA** (Consolidated Omnibus Budget Reconciliation Act).

Before choosing either of these options for maintaining your health insurance, consider their pros and cons.

The Marketplace

The Marketplace is available to people who need health insurance and have a "qualifying life event" (for example, divorce, a change in income, pregnancy, adoption of a child, or loss of a job) outside of the annual open enrollment period that runs from November 1 to January 31. The Marketplace is a group of organizations set up to facilitate the purchase of health insurance by uninsured individuals and their dependents, and by employees of small businesses, in every state. Most Marketplace plans are private plans, and all are qualified health plans (QHP). QHPs must include items and services within at least the 10 specific categories of essential health benefits (see Chapter 15).

You can access your state's Marketplace online at HealthCare.gov or by calling 800-318-2596. When you provide the requested information to find a plan, you'll learn whether you qualify for lower costs on your monthly premiums and lower out-of-pocket costs for private insurance plans; you may also qualify for free or low-cost coverage through Medicaid or the Children's Health Insurance Program (CHIP).

COBRA

COBRA is a federal law that may allow you to pay to keep yourself and your family on your employee health insurance for a limited time (usually 18 months) after your employment ends. With COBRA, you'll have to pay the full monthly premium for your health insurance plus a small administrative fee.

How does COBRA work? Let's say your employer paid 80%, or $800, of a total monthly health insurance premium of $1,000 and you paid 20%, or $200. Once you choose the COBRA option, you'll be responsible for the entire $1,000 premium plus administrative fees. Also, if you choose COBRA, you won't be able to take advantage of any subsidies or reduce out-of-pocket costs for which you may qualify

16 Maintaining Your Insurance Coverage

using the Marketplace.

Ultimately, the choice is yours, but choose wisely. If your COBRA coverage expires, you still have the option to choose a Marketplace plan.

Going without Insurance

The ACA requires you to have health insurance coverage for yourself and your dependents. Why not go without insurance? Beyond the obvious dangers of not being able to pay for healthcare out of pocket, the problem is that under the ACA, the US government will charge you a penalty.

The portion of the ACA that requires most US citizens and lawful permanent residents (see next paragraph) to have health insurance—and to be charged a penalty if without insurance—is called the "individual mandate." The penalty is considered a tax, and Congress has the right to impose a tax on US citizens. So most individuals and their dependents must have "minimum essential coverage," which includes individual market policies, job-based coverage, Medicare, Medicaid, CHIP, TRICARE (military healthcare system), and certain other coverage (for example, state health benefits risk pool, recognized by the secretary of Health and Human Services [HHS]).

What if you are not a citizen? If you plan to become a US citizen and are a lawful permanent resident (LPR) of the United States, you are still required under the ACA to purchase health insurance or face a penalty. The ACA has a lot of names for noncitizens: an LPR—that is, a permanent resident alien, resident alien permit holder, or green card holder—is anyone who resides in the United States under legally recognized and lawfully recorded permanent residence as an immigrant, and who is not a US citizen. LPRs can get health insurance through their jobs or through the Marketplace in their state of residence. Only immigrants who are lawfully present in the United States can purchase health insurance through the Marketplace. Lawful permanent residents, or qualified non-citizens, may qualify for lower costs on monthly premiums and lower out-of-pocket costs based on their income.

Some people are not required to have healthcare coverage; they are exempt for various reasons. These include people with a religious exemption, US citizens not living in the States, non-US citizens living in the States and any US possession (for example, Guam), and people who are incarcerated. Additional exceptions include members of Native American tribes; people without coverage for less than three months; people whose contribution (premium) would exceed 8% of their income; people whose income falls below the federal income tax filing threshold; and people who receive a hardship waiver from the HHS secretary.

If you choose not to buy health insurance that qualifies as minimum essential coverage, and you do not meet the eligibility requirements of age, disability, or income for Medicare or Medicaid, you could face a penalty for failure to have health insurance for more than three months. This penalty is called the "individual shared responsibility payment."

The amount of the penalty you could pay is based on the length of time you are uninsured. If your uninsured status is temporary, for six months for example, then you'll pay for just the part of the year you are uninsured. And you don't have to pay a penalty under some circumstances, though: you may qualify for an exemption if you fall under hardship exemption status, where health insurance would cost more than 8% of your household income; or you are a member of a recognized religious sect with religious objections to insurance, including Social Security and Medicare. For a list of other reasons you may not have to pay the penalty, see HealthCare.gov or call 800-318-2596.

ASSISTANCE PROGRAMS

What if you can't afford the expensive premiums and other payments associated with the Marketplace or COBRA, and you don't qualify for public assistance like Medicaid or Medicare? You can work with your

HTC social worker or reimbursement specialist to find assistance programs, including the ones listed here that help pay premiums and other costs.

Public Assistance Programs

Supplemental Security Income (SSI) and Social Security Disability Income (SSDI). These are provided by Social Security and are the largest federal programs providing assistance to people with disabilities. SSI pays monthly benefits to families with low incomes and limited assets that can be liquidated. Children with hemophilia may qualify for SSI if they meet the SSI definition of disabled, and if their family income and assets are low. SSDI is a social insurance program that offers Social Security tax benefits through your employer. If you are disabled, you can receive benefits based on your earnings.

Title V Children with Special Healthcare Needs Programs (CSHCNP). Each state has special programs under Title V government funding. Your state health department can supply more information about these programs.

Confusing? It can be! When you need instant, personalized advice on accessing state and federal assistance and entitlement programs, call Advocating for Chronic Conditions, Entitlements and Social Services (A.C.C.E.S.S.) at 888-700-7010.[1]

Private Assistance Programs

Manufacturer Copay Assistance Programs. Many factor manufacturers offer copay assistance for patients using their products who are on private insurance plans. Check with your factor manufacturer to learn about copay and other patient assistance programs.

Patient Services, Inc. (PSI). This nonprofit organization, founded by a person with hemophilia, is registered in all 50 states. PSI operates as a safety net to help maintain coverage by paying premiums and copays to qualified applicants with chronic disorders for a limited time while they transition from one policy to another. PSI assists with premium payments for patients who can't afford them, and helps patients locate health insurance. PSI services are free.[2]

Research trials. Check with your HTC for new research studies that may offer free factor concentrate to study participants.

Free trial programs. To entice customers to switch products, factor manufacturers have recently begun offering free factor through special programs. Some programs require you to make a request through your HTC; others can ship product directly to you. Check your factor manufacturer's website to see if the company offers such a program. Supplies will be limited.

Compassionate care programs. Pharmaceutical and home care companies sometimes offer compassionate care programs, also called manufacturer product assistance programs, which provide free factor to families who can prove financial hardship. Your HTC social worker can help you with this resource, or you can visit the pharmaceutical or home care websites.[3]

The entire hemophilia community—patients, HTC staff, home care companies, pharmaceutical companies—realizes that insurance is the foundation of good healthcare. Strive to maintain your current insurance, and know your options when you change insurance. If you lose insurance, know the safety nets available to you. Preparation is your best hope for preventing the disastrous situation of no insurance and no options. The waters of hemophilia insurance are choppy, full of obstacles that can shipwreck you. Navigate these waters with the help of all the resources listed here. An entire community is waiting to assist you!

Maintaining Your Insurance Coverage
Chapter 16 Summary

- When you lose your health insurance, there are two ways to maintain your coverage: the Marketplace and COBRA.
- You may qualify for public assistance or entitlement programs. When you apply for a Marketplace plan, you'll find out if you qualify for either program.
- Along with public assistance programs, investigate Supplemental Security Income (SSI) and Social Security Disability Income (SSDI).
- PSI offers temporary free insurance premium and copay coverage to qualified individuals, so you can stay insured while you work through insurance transition or loss.
- There are many ways to get free factor: research trials, free trial programs, copay assistance programs, and compassionate care services.
- When insurance change threatens or occurs, contact your HTC social worker or local hemophilia chapter.

17

Adolescence and Beyond

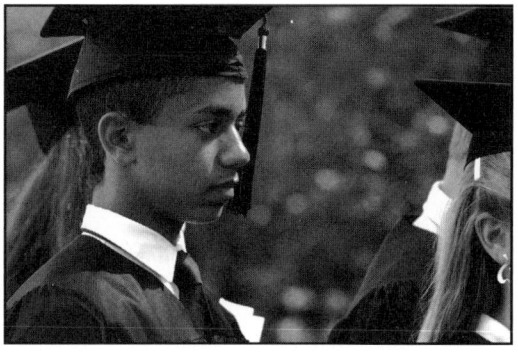

Let your child take control. You've been educating and empowering him his whole life. Now is the time to let him start making his own decisions. It's hard, especially when he makes a decision like stopping prophylaxis, but as long as these are not life-threatening issues, he needs to be able to have control and independence. —Deborah Murray, New York

At the beginning of this book, you watched your toddler start down the road toward independence. Now that road has become a highway, and your teenager will want to cruise or even race down it. Perhaps you've prepared him: helping him learn his strengths and limitations, including him in the treatment decision-making process, and letting him explore various activities. All this preparation has produced a teenager who is probably more mature than most, and who takes hemophilia seriously. Right?

You may be in for a surprise. Despite all your preparation, adolescence can bring such striking changes that you may wonder if this teen is the same child you so lovingly raised and carefully instructed. Teenagers with hemophilia, like all teenagers, show some common traits that stem from a dramatic change in physiology, a broadening social base, and a relentless desire to be independent.

Be sensitive to your teen's changing physical, social, and emotional needs. This can help you survive the turbulent years, and can help your teen mature. Your goal is to encourage him to be independent and responsible and avoid taking needless personal risks.

BIOLOGICAL CHANGES

The distinct biological, chemical, and physical differences between males and females are obvious in adolescence. Biological changes can be quick and dramatic, as your child seems to transform before your eyes. In adolescence, a boy's testosterone levels jump by 800%. Testosterone is the hormone that turns boys into men.[1] It stimulates facial hair growth and boosts muscle mass. It fuels aggression, energy, and of course, the desire to mate. The intense hormonal changes that develop your son's body into a man's body can also cause lots of stress and upheaval in his brain and nervous system. No wonder teens can be moody, defensive, withdrawn, and argumentative!

When you observe emotional or behavioral changes in your teen, try to keep in mind what's happening in his bloodstream. Along with infusions of factor, he'll be receiving continual "infusions" of testosterone—reflected in his behavior. Your job is to help him understand these physiological changes and learn to manage his emotions and behavior.

Don't forget that by the time your child is a teenager, you might be undergoing your own biological changes. Are you approaching 40? 50? Your hormones, metabolism, and appearance are all changing. Your metabolism slows down just as your teen's is revving up. Country music suddenly sounds pleasing, but your teen just discovered heavy metal. You seek peace and quiet, but your testosterone-charged teen is looking for some action. You want to continue traditional family activities or vacations, but your teen wants freedom, even though he loves his family.

Biological and psychological changes can lead to problems in communication and family dynamics; this in turn may impact hemophilia management and your child's health. Let's examine some of the ways that adolescence affects your teen with hemophilia.

INDEPENDENCE, PRIVACY, AND SECRECY

Spencer is a typical teen. He is on the pendulum that swings between the threshold of childhood sanctuary and adolescent sovereignty. He often seeks the solitude of his room, where he listens to loud music, plays video games, and talks to friends on the phone. But at bedtime, he changes back into our affectionate son, who still looks forward to our nightly ritual of talking about his day, followed by prayers, then good night hugs and kisses. —Andrea Brill, North Carolina

A teen's primary emotional need is independence: a goal he has been striving toward since he first learned to stand. Your teen may begin to separate from his family. To separate emotionally, he may need to separate physically. He may withdraw, talk less, and stay in his bedroom more. He may prefer to hang out with friends, not family. He also will—and should—demand privacy. His bedroom door is closed, his diary hidden or locked, and warning signs posted. Why? He's creating a buffer: a neutral zone where he can relax, experiment, and protect his fragile, developing personality without challenge or criticism. If he demands privacy to the point of secrecy, this may worry you. It's hard for you to respect his privacy when you believe he's not yet mature enough to make medically sound decisions.

When your teen withdraws, you'll have to learn to let go a bit and give him the space he needs. It helps to voice your expectations while acknowledging his needs. There are limits to the kind of behavior you will accept; but where can you be flexible? How can you both compromise? For example, attending a family reunion may be nonnegotiable, but attending his sibling's school play can be optional. Perhaps he no longer needs to tell you every time he has a bleed or infuses, but he must keep a log of his infusions for hospital and insurance records. He has permission to go to the rock concert if he wears his medical ID or has a medical ID card in his wallet. Encourage his input and responsibility. Make each decision less a personal conflict—you versus him—and more a choice.

Although your teen needs space and privacy, he also needs—and occasionally resents—your advice and support. Your parenting strategies must adapt, just as he is adapting. Asking questions works better than lecturing. Modeling is better than preaching. Trusting him to make decisions is better than handing down directives.

Although you need to grant him privacy, privacy can be dangerous when it becomes secrecy, especially if he spends excessive time with peers or on the Internet, at the expense of family interactions. A teen who spends hours or days withdrawn from his family may learn about relationships, privacy, and communication in inappropriate or unhealthy ways. The Internet is particularly seductive. Websites encourage teens to share personal information and to solve problems with online friends they have never met in person. Be sure to monitor your teen's time, and look over his shoulder occasionally. The danger isn't just online predators; your teen needs to develop healthy relationships with others *in person*, not solely through electronic means.

17 Adolescence and Beyond

SELF-IMAGE AND DENIAL

Concern about self-image peaks during adolescence, a time of intense self-scrutiny, self-criticism, and experimentation with looks. Even teens with no medical problems or disabilities, and who fit accepted physical norms, can be hypercritical of their bodies and abilities. Because he has hemophilia, your teen may suddenly find things to dislike about himself. He may view himself negatively because he feels different, has limits, and is still dependent on you.

Your teen may consider hemophilia a liability when forming friendships. Hemophilia is an "imperfection" that makes him different, and teens don't easily tolerate differences. Some teenagers hide hemophilia from their peers, especially when dating. Sometimes a teen even blames his parents: you "gave" him hemophilia, so it's your fault that he's unhappy with his self-image.

Your teen may be crushed when it truly hits him that hemophilia is forever, until a cure is found. A preschooler has no concern for past or future; and a school-aged child may know hemophilia is forever but, being a concrete thinker, rarely looks far into the future. As a more advanced thinker, your teen may imagine scenarios in which hemophilia makes life difficult: dating, high school sports, getting a job, health insurance, marriage.

If a teen denies his differences and tries to be just like his peers, he may deny his bleeds. Some teens hide hemophilia successfully and manage to discreetly infuse when needed, so no one ever knows. But serious denial can lead to neglect, when a teen ignores bleeds, won't infuse to stop a bleed, or refuses to wear protective gear to prevent bleeds.

You can start early to help your child accept and tolerate his hemophilia. Don't hide it, but don't make it the defining point of his life. Let him decide when and who to tell about his hemophilia.[2] Try to keep his disorder in perspective. Give him these messages:

- What's important is not what happens to us in our lives, it's what we do about what happens to us.
- Hemophilia isn't the reason that good or bad things happen, and it's never a reason to limit our enjoyment of life.
- Our differences are what make us special.

From the start, show your child that everyone's differences should be respected, tolerated, and appreciated.

RISK-TAKING BEHAVIOR

With his boundless energy, pumping testosterone, natural sense of invulnerability, and desire for independence, a teen with hemophilia will want to push his limits.

Some risk taking is actually healthy. Moving to a new city, making new friends, starting a business, breaking with tradition—all these risks involve some anxiety or fear but can bring immense rewards. Learning new skills means taking risks. For example, thrilling activities like rock climbing or whitewater rafting carry risks of injury; auditioning for a part in a play carries a risk of rejection. But new skills offer the chance to achieve, experience, and build character. Challenging the body and mind stimulates growth. When challenged, a teen can discover his strengths and limitations, and he can learn to be responsible for his actions.

How can you safely encourage risk taking? Recommend activities that occur in a healthy, structured environment, preferably with an adult mentor. Sports are one obvious way: baseball, basketball, skiing, and martial arts all provide plenty of risk under safe conditions with experienced adults. Or enroll your teen in driver's education classes. Nothing is more exciting than getting his license! Help your teen choose activities that offer the opportunity to hear, "That's safe, but only when . . ." instead of, "No, that's not safe; you'll get hurt." Translate that last comment into teen-speak, and he hears, "I don't trust you to be competent and learn." When he has positive outlets for adventure and risk, your teen will build his sense of accomplishment, control, and confidence.

If your teen is not prepared or guided, his actions may become dangerous, particularly if he doesn't accept his hemophilia. He may rebel against parental restrictions. He may seek approval from his peers for risky behavior. He may try to seize control of a life too rigidly structured by adults. If this happens, the same activities that could challenge him, test his endurance, and build maturity may cause injury or permanent damage.

Of course, some rebellious or experimental activities should never be attempted, regardless of hemophilia. High-speed driving, drinking and driving, and drugs are real dangers to our youths. It's well known that by middle school, over 10% of students may be experimenting with marijuana, alcohol, or even hash. By grade 12, more than 30% of them are regularly smoking illegal substances or drinking.[3] Some illegal drugs, often bought on school playgrounds, are being mixed with common household poisons, so a teen may not know what toxins he is inhaling, ingesting, or injecting.

Why do teens take dangerous risks? Sometimes it's curiosity, sometimes peer pressure. Unhealthy risk taking can also be a reaction to overprotective parents. Years of limiting and monitoring your child's behavior may leave him feeling frustrated and helpless. He wants to make up for lost time. The greater the degree of parental overprotection, the more teens may want to push the envelope and engage in risky behavior.

On the other hand, a lot of parental control may have the opposite effect. Teens may give up trying to take control of their activities, lives, and decisions. Allow your teen some freedom and responsibility, including the freedom to choose activities, which may mean taking risks. Prepare him by reviewing safety rules. You'll encourage the confidence and self-esteem he needs to take more control of his life as he matures.

ENCOURAGING RESPONSIBILITY AND INDEPENDENCE

Children with hemophilia depend on their parents for a time, like all children. Eventually, they learn to go to the bathroom by themselves, feed themselves, tie their shoes, and brush their teeth. And eventually, they learn when and how to infuse. Your goal is to decrease your teen's dependency, increase his sense of competence, and enhance his sense of responsibility. You can do this in many ways:

Allow your child to make his own decisions. Begin at age three or four, when safety is not an issue. Teach him how to detect bleeds. Help him understand the consequences of untreated bleeds and of his behavior. Tell him which activities will benefit his body and which will hurt. Show faith in his judgment. Instead of, "It looks to me like you're having a bleed. Let's get some factor," try saying, "Do you think you're having a bleed? Will you tell me when you need factor?"

Introduce your teen to other teens with hemophilia. Your teen may be less likely to hide hemophilia when he knows he belongs to a community that supports him.[4] He'll meet adults with hemophilia who can model success, involvement, and responsibility.

Educate your teen about risk-taking behaviors. Drinking causes loss of inhibition, which may lead to more risk-taking behavior, such as speeding. Examine your state's website for laws and consequences regarding drinking, driving, and sex.[5]

Pick your battles carefully. Hair may not be the hill to die on when your teen shaves his head or decides to have dreadlocks. Decide which behaviors are nonnegotiable, and then involve your teen in making rules for the rest. What time does he suggest for curfew? Then negotiate. Show respect for his opinion—*even if you choose not to follow it*. Reexamine and modify your rules when your child's capabilities grow and he matures. When possible, limit nonnegotiable rules to those that endanger physical and emotional safety.

Expect your teen to self-infuse. He can learn through his HTC or home care company. He should be independently infusing himself as a teen, with little or no help from you. He's also capable of ordering his own factor. Give him phone numbers and product information, and walk him through his first order.

Expect rebellion. View his rebellion as a developmental milestone, a necessary rite of passage. To your teen, rebellion can be an opportunity to express himself and to dialogue with you. Expect him to challenge and test rules concerning hemophilia and non-hemophilia issues. But don't take it too personally. His rebellion is more about him than about you—he is growing up.

It's not always easy. Even children who are desperate to be independent suddenly turn around and say, "I can't. *You* do it."

Here's some great childrearing advice: Don't do anything for your children that they can safely do for themselves. When you teach your child to be independent, you're not only teaching him how to manage his life, you're implicitly saying, "I respect your intelligence and abilities. You know best when you are having a bleed. You're able to care for yourself. You are competent."

TAKING OWNERSHIP: HIS BODY, HIS HEMOPHILIA

To help your teen accept more personal responsibility, give him a sense of ownership of his body: his body belongs to him, and his actions directly affect his health. Previously, you acted as his caretaker. You checked for bleeds, administered factor, called doctors, made appointments, ordered supplies, talked to HTC staff, logged infusions, and selected his factor brand. Which of these tasks can he now do?

He can do most of them. Train him, step by step, to take ownership. When he asks you to infuse him because he's tired—and he knows how to do it, isn't in severe pain, isn't disabled—*just say no*. Consider allowing him to suffer the physical consequences. Eventually, he'll learn that his parents won't bail him out because he doesn't feel like infusing, or it's late, or he's in a hurry.

Taking ownership also means considering the safety of current teen trends, such as piercings and tattoos. Your teen needs to know about the obvious risks of tissue or blood infection, and know if he needs to infuse beforehand. Depending on your state of residence, after age 18 or 21, he is legally able to get piercings or tattoos without your permission. Before then, you have some control over what he does to his body. Decide what's acceptable in your family. Discuss piercings, tattoos, hairstyles, and clothing choices *before* they become problematic or irreversible.

Ownership means that your teen must be proactive in nourishing his body. It's hard to eat healthy in our American culture of fast food and sedentary lifestyles. Many teens spend huge chunks of time playing video games online, watching television, or texting. On average, American teens weigh more than their parents did at this age, and obesity is rampant (see Chapter 11). Encourage fresh foods, cut down on soft drinks, and get your teen moving!

You may notice that your child's sleep patterns change dramatically when he becomes an adolescent. Some teens sleep until noon, and others cut back on sleep. A minimum of eight hours is ideal to allow the mind to rest and recharge. Staying online late at night makes it hard to unwind and go to sleep, yet this is when many teens love to surf. Try setting a nightly Internet curfew for the whole family, to encourage better sleep and to spend quality time together.

> **Checklist: Topics to Discuss with Your Teen**
>
> - Internet usage: how often, how much, sharing private information online
> - Driving: permit, driver's education, license, rules of the road, seatbelts, DUI
> - Sex: education, morals, birth control, responsibility, STDs
> - Drugs: types, peer pressure, legal consequences, health consequences, addiction
> - School: grades, college preparation, extracurricular activities
> - Peers: choice of friends, social activities, dating
> - Spirituality: personal beliefs, family beliefs, tolerance
> - Hemophilia: prophy, diagnosing bleeds, dosing, HTC visits, self-infusion, ordering factor, logging infusions
> - Work: finding first job, work ethics, insurance
> - Health: eating well, sleep habits, excercise, nutrition
> - Risk taking: appropriate activities, dangerous choices, reasons why
> - Emotions: depression, anxiety, sleep issues, relationships

TRANSITION: ADOLESCENCE TO ADULTHOOD

Your child's adolescence seems to fly by as he becomes more independent and active. Before you know it, he's 18 and ready to strike out on his own. You'll probably help him practice for his driver's license test, submit college applications, celebrate proms and graduation, enroll in the Selective Service System[6] (even a teen with a medical disorder like hemophilia must at least enroll), and apply for jobs. Parents of 18-year-olds often say, "I can't *believe* how fast the time went!"

It pays to prepare. Here's a list of the main transitions your child will master, and each associated age:

Transition Event	Approximate Age
Driver's permit	16+
Driver's license	16-17
SATs or ACTs (college entrance exams)	16-17
College applications	17-18
High school graduation	17-18
Select Service System registration	18
Health insurance changes	26+

HEALTH INSURANCE CHANGES

Parents often overlook changes in health insurance, a key transition. It's easier to overlook it, now that your teen won't cap out, be turned down for insurance for a preexisting condition, and can stay on your insurance until he's 26. Eventually, he'll need to land a job with health benefits.

Don't wait until your child is 26 to learn about his options. Start when he's 14 or 15. Speak to your factor provider, HTC social worker, or insurance company. Begin teaching your child about your policy and how his care is covered. Remember that of all the transitions you both face in the teen years, *health insurance coverage is the most important*.

TRANSITIONING TO ADULT HTCS

If your HTC allows it, your teen can keep the same hematologist and comprehensive HTC team he had as a pediatric patient. But in many cases, when he turns 18, he'll be transitioned to the adult hematology department. Your teen's social worker can help with this transition, and may even stay on as his social worker.

The needs of 18-year-olds with hemophilia differ from those of younger teens. By age 18, most hemophilia patients are self-infusing, working or attending college, and ready to accept total personal responsibility for their care, including ordering factor.

Perhaps the biggest change is that your teen is seen at the HTC alone. Patient confidentiality is key. Your teen will be expected to give his own medical history and speak directly to his hematologist and social worker. He'll need to share information about his sex life, to prevent disease and unwanted pregnancy. He'll be asked about drug and alcohol use, nutrition, career planning, and insurance.

It's truly hard for some parents to accept their child's independence. At the HTC, you are no longer privileged to know all about his private life. Take courage from the fact that the professional, experienced team at your HTC will advise and monitor him well. You may be consulted as needed, but if all goes well, you'll have only a small role in his ongoing healthcare.

CAREER CHOICES

If you want your child to grow into a truly independent adult, you need to think seriously and early about his employment so you can give him practical advice. His career choice can affect not only his health and happiness, but more important, his insurance. Begin in early high school to help him start thinking about job choices and interests.

Consider his health first. Manual labor like construction is hard on joints and muscles, and may require frequent infusions. Yet as they enter adulthood, some teens are weaned off prophylaxis, and even those on prophylaxis may experience breakthrough bleeding. For most people with hemophilia, heavy manual labor is unrealistic as a career. But even the field of manual labor can still be open to him; for example, he could work in construction management instead of ground operations.

Next, you and your teen should consider career inclination, level of job satisfaction, and general happiness. What are his interests and skills? Job satisfaction is based on enjoyment, challenge, and a sense of competence and contribution, not just job security or financial reward. Introduce your teen to a variety of activities that challenge his skills: chemistry, music, art, medicine, writing, engineering, travel, acting–the list is endless! Your child will discover his skills and passions.

Choice of employment will directly affect medical insurance coverage. Good coverage is essential for someone with hemophilia. Working for the government provides excellent coverage. Large companies, banks, and hospitals also offer a wide range of coverage. Private companies, self-employment, and small firms may provide less coverage. When possible, your son should get a copy of a prospective employer's insurance policy before accepting a job, and have it examined by a social worker who is familiar with insurance as it applies to hemophilia.

> **Alternatives to College**
>
> Not all young adults want to attend college, and not all can afford college. There are many alternatives to college: family businesses, clerical positions, trade schools specializing in technical careers. Many scholarship programs exist just for students with hemophilia who wish to attend college or trade school (see www.kelleycom.com). Work with your child's high school to find volunteer opportunities or summer jobs that offer experience in different careers. Working with children, working in an office, coaching sports, working in retail sales, and professional internships can all open doors to a bright future.

When your child finds an appropriate job with good medical coverage, he'll need to decide what to tell his employer. If hemophilia affects his job performance, through absences or inability to do heavy labor, he should consider informing his employer about his hemophilia. If his job is flexible, he might be able to make up hours outside his regular shift. It's a tough decision: He may risk discrimination if he reveals his hemophilia too early. He may face resentment if he reveals it too late, after many job absences.

Prophylaxis will have a tremendous positive influence on securing and keeping jobs. If your teen stops prophy, he may still be in excellent condition for work, because his joints will be preserved. If he can continue prophylaxis, then his range of job opportunities widens because his bleeds are prevented.

LOVING ENOUGH TO LET GO

Adolescence is a time of tremendous transition. It may feel like the earth's tectonic plates under your house have rumbled, then shifted, and left behind a smoldering rubble of emotions, dirty dishes, and laundry. But remember that this is natural and inevitable. It's even a sign of your parenting success. Yes, you've done a good job!

When raising children, we often forget the most fundamental fact: *It's your child's goal in life to successfully become independent of you.* It's easy to forget this goal when you're engrossed in daily life.

Independence. It's the path your child started down when he first learned to walk. It's the pride that surges when he scores a goal or makes black belt. It's the glow he feels when he does his first infusion. It's the thrill he experiences when he gets his driver's license. Independence is the new horizon he spies when he sets off to college or his first job. You can help him travel to that horizon if you start when he's young. Help your little ones make good decisions by setting them up for success, with choices that encourage positive outcomes. Success builds on success, and with each success, your child's self-esteem grows. Yours will too, especially when he's ready to leave home, confident, healthy, and educated about hemophilia. He'll feel mature and positive, and he'll appreciate all your efforts, sacrifice, and love through the years. Good luck!

Adolescence and Beyond
Chapter 17 Summary

- As a teen's physiology undergoes dramatic changes, his emotional needs and behaviors change. His primary emotional need is independence.
- When a teen with hemophilia feels he is different, has limits, and still depends on his parents, his self-image might be affected.
- Teens feel invincible and may deny their hemophilia by ignoring bleeds, refusing infusions, or refusing to wear proper safety equipment.
- Teens can take some risks in a healthy, structured environment, preferably with an adult mentor.
- Some risk-taking behaviors are never acceptable, including high-speed driving, drinking and driving, unprotected sex, and illegal drugs.
- Expect rebellion against hemophilia and non-hemophilia issues. View his rebellion as an outlet for self-expression and learning.
- Transition means that your teen is preparing for adulthood: driver's license, graduation, first job, Selective Service System registration, college entrance exams, college applications, adult HTC.
- Prepare your teen for an independent future by examining college and vocational training options. Help him prepare for exams, help him find out what he can do well, and investigate scholarships in the hemophilia community.

Conclusion

An Invincible Summer

In the depth of winter, I finally learned that there was in me an invincible summer. —Albert Camus

I began writing the first edition of this book when my son was only 18 months old, in 1989. It seemed a way to manage my own fears, to educate myself when no resources were available. When he'd been diagnosed with hemophilia at age one month, I was just 30—a new mother, scared and tearful. Before his birth, I had firmly planned my life. My ego was reaping the rewards of a carefully constructed career. I felt that I was in control, on top of the world. Children would complete the vision I projected in my mind. But destiny set another path for me. Hemophilia shattered my plans, upset my confidence in the faith on which I was raised, and stirred deep self-doubts. Why me? Why this child? Could I handle this? For me, hemophilia resurrected disturbing but fundamental questions about human suffering. Suffering, it suddenly seemed, was everywhere.

Psychiatrist Elisabeth Kübler-Ross wrote, "You will not grow if you sit in a beautiful flower garden, but you will grow if you are sick, if you are in pain, if you experience losses, and if you do not put your head in the sand, but take the pain as a gift to you with a very, very specific purpose."

My garden of beautiful dreams froze as an emotional winter set in. At first, like many parents with a newly diagnosed child, all I could do was shiver and hunker down. But here was my ultimate choice as a parent: to be overwhelmed by pain, or to do something with it. As I read about hemophilia, and as my son endured my laborious learning curve, I wondered how I could at least make his pain count for something. What if I shared our experiences with others, so no other parent would have to repeat my ignorant blunders? As I gathered parenting tidbits from other hemophilia families, I was also eager to share their knowledge with a wider community. It seemed that we were all groping in the dark, waiting for light. For me, a personal mission was born.

This mission has become my lifelong journey. I never dreamed that all this would happen, but my work has continued to expand through the years. My company now donates educational materials and millions of dollars in factor annually to developing countries. My personal mission was founded on the day I consciously chose to reject hemophilia as the darkness of a terrible winter. Instead, I chose to bask—even sweat—in a bright summer of personal growth.

Perhaps one of the most enduring and challenging tasks many of us face is to discover our life's mission. Having a child with hemophilia causes most parents to ponder life's suffering, meaning, and purpose. Some ask, "Why was I put on this earth?" Others ask, "What can I do with my life to make a difference?"

Perhaps you'll find purpose in the pain. Perhaps you can frame hemophilia in your own life as more than a chronic disorder. Could it be a special gift? Could it offer a chance to discover your own life's mission? Could it be your path to personal development? Think about how much you've grown since you heard the diagnosis, and what you've learned. What has your child brought that you might never have known without hemophilia? One mother reflected, "Even the darkest moments turn out to be okay. You become stronger, and your child does as well."

I hope that after reading *Raising a Child with Hemophilia*, you'll have the tools you need to begin building your life with hemophilia. And more than that, I hope you'll discover the rare gift of purpose. I hope you'll find confidence knowing that life with hemophilia is not only manageable, but also joyful and rewarding. Yes, your beautiful garden doesn't look exactly like you planned it. But there is so much you can do to adapt, so much you can learn! Your days of tears will

Conclusion

become days of triumph. Winter gives way to summer. There is very little that your child with hemophilia—and you—won't be able to conquer.

As I complete this fifth edition, my three children are all adults embarking on their own lives. At 59, I find myself straddling this moment in my life, looking backward and forward. Although I've accomplished many things, my mission constantly beckons. I look forward to the future and all its seasons, with joy and gratitude.

Don't squander what could be a rare gift. Accept with gratitude the lessons you're learning. Then share what you learn, practically and personally, as a gift to others. You can help your child find purpose through pain, find his own mission using a positive mindset. Show him that summer can eclipse winter.

Above all, love your child as no one else can. Love and respect yourself, too, for you are raising this child. Hemophilia will change your life and challenge you to venture out from the security of a beautiful garden. But on this unexpected journey of personal discovery, through harsh terrain, find your invincible summer inside. You can make hemophilia a positive turning point in your life, prompting you to discover hidden talents, greater compassion, deeper connections, and a higher purpose.

> We are blessed. We have two beautiful, healthy, happy boys, and we love them no matter what. I used to wonder, "Why me?" But now I think, "Why not me?" I can handle it. This is the life chosen for me, and I love my life! —Karen Ward, Maine

Notes

1 "Your child has hemophilia."

1. Elisabeth Kübler-Ross, MD. *On Death and Dying*. (New York: Touchstone Press, 1969).

2. Sadness is a normal reaction to life's unexpected blows. When sadness persists for weeks, even months, and interferes with normal activities that used to give you joy, you could be suffering from depression. Some sadness, often called "baby blues," is experienced by up to 80% of women who have recently given birth. Postpartum depression is more serious and can affect between 5% and 25% of women after childbirth. The diagnosis of hemophilia can further impact women who are already suffering mild to severe depression. Please speak to a social worker, clergy, or licensed therapist to determine if you are depressed. Depression can and should be treated.

3. In 67% of hemophilia cases, there is a family history. The other 33% happen spontaneously, with no family history. In spontaneous cases, the **genetic mutation** may occur in the mother (she is a carrier) or in the child (he has hemophilia and his mother is not a carrier).

4. Locate the nearest HTC by calling NHF at 800-42-HANDI to request a list of national centers, or visit the US Centers for Disease Control and Prevention (CDC) website for a list: www.cdc.gov.

5. Although a hematologist is a blood specialist, most are trained to be oncologists (cancer doctors) and few are bleeding disorder specialists. A hematologist may have little training in hemophilia and may never have treated a person with hemophilia. Hematologists associated with HTCs are bleeding disorder specialists experienced with, and trained in, hemophilia.

6. Warning: A feeling common to new parents is anxiety at hearing more experienced parents share their most traumatic stories. It's natural to want to share how we have triumphed, survived, and become stronger parents. But new parents should be eased gently into their new life with hemophilia with stories that do not frighten them.

2 What Is Hemophilia?

1. Hemophilia A occurs in about 1 in 5,000 live male births. Hemophilia B occurs in about 1 in 20,000 live male births. According to the CDC, the exact number of people living with hemophilia in the United States is unknown. At the time of this writing, the number of people with hemophilia in the United States is estimated at about 20,000, based on expected births and deaths since 1994. http://www.cdc.gov/ncbddd/hemophilia/data.html (accessed Nov. 8, 2015).

2. It is possible for someone to get hemophilia later in life; this is an autoimmune condition called **acquired hemophilia**.

3. Blood clotting is one of the most complex body processes. A great way for you, your child, your relatives, and school staff to learn the basics of blood clotting is to read some children's books: *They'll Probably Ask You . . . What Is Hemophilia?* and *Tell Them the Facts!* by Laureen A. Kelley; *A Drop of Blood* by Paul Showers. See Appendix A.

4. VWD is a deficiency of the protein called von Willebrand factor. VWD affects platelet function and sometimes factor VIII levels. To learn more, read *A Guide to Living with von Willebrand Disease* by Laureen A. Kelley. See Appendix A.

5. Technically, the differences among severity levels relate to the activity level of the factor, not to its absence. Your child may actually have a normal amount of factor, but because most of it is inactive, the blood does not clot well.

6. Learn more about prophylaxis in Chapter 7.

7. Carriers whose factor levels are between 40% and 60% may show unusual bleeding tendencies

after trauma. Many carriers have factor levels below 50% and have regular bleeding; they are called symptomatic carriers, which really means that they have mild hemophilia.

8. It's also possible for a mother to carry a defective gene in only a few of her eggs, without having the defective gene in the rest of the cells in her body. This condition is called mosaicism (or gonadal mosaicism, or germ line mosaicism, referring to the eggs). A woman who is a genetic mosaic would not show up as a carrier on carrier tests, even though she may give birth to one or more boys with hemophilia. There is no way to test how many of a woman's eggs carry the hemophilia gene.

3 The First Few Months

1. See Paul Clement, "Just A Snip? The Circumcision Decision," *PEN*, Aug. 2015. Download a free copy from LA Kelley Communications, www.kelleycom.com/archives.html.

2. Of the world's male population, 70% are uncircumcised ("Male Circumcision: Global Trends and Determinants of Prevalence, Safety and Acceptability." World Health Organization: 2007. www.who.int). Most circumcisions are part of the religious rituals of Judaism or Islam. Currently, circumcision for religious reasons is safe when performed with prophylactic infusions and prescribed follow-up treatments. Always consult your HTC first.

3. To treat these bleeds, your child will need to be verbal and tell you he feels tingling or bleeding.

4. See Chapter 5 for a discussion of mouth bleeds.

5. Amicar is effective in people with severe hemophilia *only* after a dose of factor.

6. A sign is medical evidence of disease (objective.) A symptom is a medical concern that only the patient can feel (subjective).

7. A swollen tongue or face may occur as an allergic or anaphylactic reaction to factor or food. If your child has a swollen face and any kind of respiratory distress such as wheezing or trouble breathing, call 911. A bleed may not progress quickly, but anaphylaxis will. Anaphylaxis doesn't have to happen immediately after eating a food. It can happen any time up to 48 hours after exposure to the allergen.

8. Head bleeds are not easy for a hematologist to diagnose, and 95% of early head bleeds are not detected by computed tomography (CT) scans, which are usually ordered by doctors when a bleed is suspected.

4 The Doctor-Parent Partnership

1. Hematologists also treat patients with cancer and leukemia. If your hematologist is not part of an HTC, he or she may not be familiar enough with hemophilia to adequately diagnose certain bleeds. This could mean that your child may not receive proper treatment. Find out how much experience your hematologist has with hemophilia.

2. Most interns start their residency in July. If you visit the ER in July, ask if the attending physician is newly graduated, and don't hesitate to ask for someone with more experience.

3. For example, a CT scan of the head is equivalent to the radiation exposure of 20 chest x-rays. If your physician orders a CT scan for every head bump, this cumulative exposure may represent a significant lifetime risk. Read Paul Clement, "CT Scans for Head Bumps: Always the Best Choice?" *PEN*, May 2011 (www.kelleycom.com).

4. Needle sizes increase inversely to their numbers: a 23-gauge needle is larger than a 25-gauge needle.

5. Arteries should never be used, unless a hematologist is consulted and recommends it when no other venous access is available.

Notes

6. It's always a good idea to bring the factor that is shipped to you at home through your factor provider (see Chapter 6) because most community hospitals do not stock factor or may not stock your particular brand or dose.

7. Some ER policies will not allow infusion of drugs mixed beforehand or mixed by parents without supervision. Check the policy before you arrive. Medical staff mixing factor for the first time often shake the vial to help "dissolve" factor—a common mistake. Never shake the reconstituting factor, as this may cause some of it to foam, effectively decreasing the dose.

5 The First Year

1. Always closely supervise a child in a walker. Doors to the cellar stairs or front and back of the house should be shut and locked. Any child, with or without hemophilia, could sustain a head injury from a tumble downstairs in his walker. Consider stationary walkers or exercisers, which pose little risk of injury.

2. Create a homemade ice pack from ice cubes in a plastic bag or thin towel, or use a packet of frozen peas. Also try reusable pediatric cold packs, available from most pharmacies or your factor provider. Be careful when using ice: leave on the skin for a maximum of 10 minutes at a time, and less time for babies. Ice can damage the skin just like frostbite.

3. Some potentially serious side effects are associated with Amicar. As with all medications, discuss its use and possible side effects with your doctor. Other medications, such as tranexamic acid, can also slow the breakdown of clots. Never give Amicar if a kidney bleed is in progress.

4. If left unattended, bleeding in the tongue may have serious consequences because the tongue is near the throat—a danger zone. See Chapter 3 for more on danger zones.

5. All head bumps should be treated seriously (see Chapter 3), regardless of your child's factor deficiency level. Always call your hematologist to discuss treatment.

6. See Appendix E for a list of medicines to avoid.

7. NSAIDs are drugs such as ibuprofen and naproxen with **analgesic**, antipyretic, and anti-inflammatory effects. They reduce pain, fever, and inflammation.

8. The MedicAlert Foundation (www.medicalert.org, 800-432-5378) has information on ordering identification tags. See Appendix B.

9. EMLA, a topical numbing cream, is a prescription product manufactured by AstraZeneca. Effective in eliminating the pain of needlesticks, it must be applied to the needlestick site for 30 to 45 minutes before the infusion. L.M.X.4 is a nonprescription topical local anesthetic manufactured by Ferndale Laboratories, Inc.

6 Becoming a Savvy Consumer

1. Payers are (1) private insurance companies, such as Blue Cross Blue Shield or Aetna, that reimburse for factor used by people who either have health insurance through their employers or purchase insurance privately; or (2) public payers, such as the federal or state government, that reimburse for factor used by people who are classified as low income (Medicaid) or are elderly or disabled (Medicare). For more on payers, see Chapter 15.

2. To encourage development of drugs for rare disorders, the FDA awards some factor concentrates orphan drug status, ensuring the manufacturer exclusive production rights for seven years and effectively eliminating competition. The orphan drug status for most current products has expired, allowing new products to enter the market and creating more choice.

3. Purity is measured in units of factor concentrate per milligram (mg) of protein. Intermediate purity products have a specific activity between 1 and 10 IU/mg of total protein. High purity concentrates have a specific activity between 10 and 150 IU/mg of total protein, and ultrapure products have a specific activity from 150 to 2,000 IU/mg of total protein.

4. Although the current products have excellent safety records, no product is 100% safe or pure.

5. Solvent-detergent washes and heat treatments are only minimally effective against non-enveloped viruses such as hepatitis A and B-19 parvovirus. See Appendix D.

6. Although not made from human blood, some recombinant products may add albumin, which comes from plasma, in the final steps of manufacturing. It's debatable why some recombinant factor concentrate brands use a viral inactivation step: possibly for marketing purposes, to appease consumers' concerns about safety. Or possibly, if the cell culture consists of mammalian cells, it might be infected by a virus that could slip past the purification process to the final product. There could also be other as yet unidentified viruses. A viral inactivation step may stop these viruses.

7. Albumin is the most abundant plasma protein, and since its first medical use in 1941, it has never been shown to transmit HIV, HBV, or HCV. Although albumin is virally inactivated, some viruses can still remain infective.

8. Always include your HTC hematologist in your decision to try a new product, preferably with his or her consent and supervision.

9. If your hospital is an HMO and sells drugs, its prices may be lower than those in a regular hospital.

10. In 1992, Congress passed the Veterans Health Care Act (VHCA), which established section 340B of the Public Health Service Act. The PHS Act allows the lowest manufacturer purchase prices on prescription outpatient drugs for certain covered entities: federally funded entities and public hospitals that treat a disproportionate share of Medicaid and Medicare patients. The intent of Congress was to stretch scarce federal resources as far as possible, while reaching more eligible patients and providing more comprehensive services. These covered entities serve special groups of patients, usually the uninsured or low income, people with catastrophic medical costs, or the underserved in the care of certain diseases, such as AIDS. Federally funded covered entities named in the VHCA include community health centers, black lung clinics, family planning centers, Native Hawaiian Health Centers, and HTCs that receive grants from the Maternal and Child Health Bureau (MCHB).

7 Prophylax—and Relax!

1. Recombinant products are recommended for prophylaxis. MASAC Recommendation Concerning Prophylaxis 179, http://www.hemophilia.org/Researchers-Healthcare-Providers/Medical-and-Scientific-Advisory-Council-MASAC/MASAC-Recommendations/MASAC-Recommendation-Concerning-Prophylaxis (accessed Nov. 8, 2015).

2. A port may be the best solution for families who want to do on-demand home infusions, live far from an HTC, or have a baby or young child with hard-to-find veins. The time spent driving to an HTC for an infusion is time spent bleeding into a joint and causing cumulative, permanent damage. A port can offer a quicker way to get factor into a baby or young child. There are many considerations when using a port (see page 122).

3. A large international study (S. C. Gouw, J. G. van der Bom, and H. M. van den Berg, "Treatment-Related Risk Factors of Inhibitor Development in Previously Untreated Patients with Hemophilia A: The CANAL Cohort Study," *Blood* 109 (2007): 4648–54.) found that prophylaxis reduced the risk of inhibitors. Prophylaxis (started at a median age of 20 months) was associated with a 60% lower risk of inhibitors as compared to on-demand treatment. Studies have also found an increased risk of inhibitors for patients receiving initial high-dose and high-frequency treatments when the immune system is on high alert (after surgery or severe bleeds requiring high-dose or prolonged treatment). It's believed that the risk can be minimized by avoiding infusions during infections or on the same day as vaccinations, and by delaying elective surgery during the first 20

days of exposure to factor, when inhibitors are most likely to develop.

4. DVT may develop with no signs or symptoms, and may go undiagnosed unless the physician specifically looks for it with a Doppler ultrasound, MRI, or CT scan. The longer the catheter is in place, the greater the risk of developing DVT. Most DVTs occur after catheters have been in place for at least four years. Some studies report a 22% to 50% rate of DVT in hemophilia patients with ports. In some cases, there are no signs or symptoms of a DVT. In other cases, a DVT may cause pain in the shoulder, neck, or arm; aching discomfort; swelling; enlarged surface veins; or discoloration on the side of the body where the thrombosis exists. If a clot breaks loose, it may travel to the lungs, blocking arterial blood supply to the lungs, possibly causing death. Notify your HTC immediately if you observe any of these signs or symptoms.

5. Applying direct pressure on a venipuncture site with a gauze pad for a full 10 minutes also minimizes scarring and allows repeated use of a vein.

6. It's critical to allow complete healing before inserting a new port.

7. Two clinical studies show the benefits of prophylactic therapy in hemophilia patients. See I. M. Nilsson, E. Berntorp, T. Lofqvist, et al., "Twenty Five Years' Experience of Prophylactic Treatment in Severe Haemophilia A and B," *Journal of Internal Medicine* 232 (1992): 25-32. See also M. Manco-Johnson, T. Abshire, A. Shapiro, et al., "Prophylaxis Versus Episodic Treatment to Prevent Joint Disease in Boys with Severe Hemophilia," *New England Journal of Medicine* 357 (6): 535-44.

9 Hemophilia at Home and on the Road

1. Remember that severity levels are based on the amount of factor active in the bloodstream. Severe is less than 1% active. Moderate is 1% to 5% active. Mild is 6% to 50% active.

2. See Chapter 7 on prophylaxis.

3. See Chapter 13 for a discussion of DDAVP.

4. See Chapter 15 on insurance.

5. See Appendix A.

6. Many sources give the location of all HTCs in the United States. Visit the CDC, NHF, or WFH websites.

7. This may not be possible if you have state-funded insurance such as Medicaid. Check with your HTC for the best way to prepare for vacations and trips.

8. When traveling overseas, you may need to bring enough factor for your entire trip. Home care companies can't ship outside the United States, and customs may not allow your family member to ship your personal medicine to you.

10 School Days

1. Don't give school personnel lengthy books. Instead, try *Tell Them the Facts!* by Laureen A. Kelley. This book for teenagers is also appropriate for adults new to hemophilia. See Appendix A. There are also PowerPoint presentations that can be downloaded online for school personnel, through NHF, HFA and a few home care companies.

2. It may not be necessary to explain the whole infusion process. This will only complicate matters, and staff may never see you do it. But be sure to review it with the school nurse later.

3. Always have your child bring a signed note to school excusing him from a particular class or activity if he is recovering from a bleed. Speak to the physical education teacher at the beginning of the school year about respecting your child's reports of a bleed.

4. Section 504 of the Rehabilitation Act of 1973 (PL 93-112) is a civil rights law that prohibits discrimination against people with disabilities in any program or activity receiving or benefiting from federal financial assistance. Google Section 504 or visit www.justice.gov for more information.

5. Always contact school officials when a student is being bullied. They are obligated by law to respond.

6. Terrence Webster-Doyle, *Why is Everybody Always Picking on Me? A Guide to Handling Bullies* (Education for Peace Publications, 1977).

11 Sports and Summer Camp

1. Michael Gurian, *The Wonder of Boys* (New York: Jeremy P. Tarcher/Putnam, 1977).

2. http://www.cdc.gov/nchs/fastats/obesity-overweight.htm

3. Eric Schlosser, *Fast Food Nation: The Dark Side of the American Meal* (Boston: Houghton Mifflin, 2001).

4. This is more than 15% of American children. http://www.cdc.gov/obesity/data/childhood.html

5. HTC staff used to teach R.I.C.E. for treatment after a bleed and an infusion: Rest, Ice, Compression, Elevation. Recently this has been criticized because rest and ice could delay healing. Please check with your HTC about what guidelines to follow after a bleed and an infusion.

6. Getting a well-fitted helmet takes some knowledge. If you've never bought a helmet for your child, get one at a specialty bike store. Bike specialists can fit the helmet to your child, showing you how to use the bits and pieces you'll need to customize it completely.

7. *Playing It Safe: Bleeding Disorders, Sports and Exercise*. Available from NHF (800-42-HANDI). See Appendix A.

8. Visit NHF's website for a list of hemophilia summer camps in the US: www.hemophilia.org

12 Family Matters

1. Read *Teach Your Child about Hemophilia* by Laureen A. Kelley. See Appendix A to order.

13 Deciding to Have More Children

1. I. Plug, E. P. Mauser-Bunschoten, et al., "Bleeding in Carriers of Hemophilia," *Blood* 108:1 (2006): 52–56.

2. Keep in mind that women's factor VIII levels may vary up to 100% as a result of hormone activity, although this is not true of factor IX levels.

3. A specific mutation, called an inversion in intron 22 (IVS 22), has been identified in 50% of samples of men with severe hemophilia A. Over 1,000 mutations causing hemophilia have been identified, and more are being identified all the time.

4. The indirect test is also known as linkage analysis, or restriction length fragment polymorphisms (RLFP).

5. High levels of estrogen and progesterone, associated with some birth control pills, will often raise a carrier's factor VIII levels enough to control bleeding problems.

6. C. H. Hsiao, H. C. Wang, et al., "Fetal Gender Screening by Ultrasound at 11 to 13(+6) Weeks," *Acta Obstetricia et Gynecologica Scandinavica* 87:1 (2008): 8–13.

7. Some sources cite an amniocentesis miscarriage risk of 1 in 200-400 women tested. Another cites a risk as low as 1 in 1,600. One large study found the rate as low as 0.06%. See K. Eddleman, "Pregnancy Loss Rates after Mid-trimester Amniocentesis," *Obstetrics and Gynecology* 108 (2006): 1067–72.

8. Although rare, ICH is serious. As the blood pools, it compresses nerves and reduces blood flow within the brain. An infant with undiagnosed ICH could suffer permanent brain damage.

9. As of this writing, experts have not identified a single, specific cause of intracranial bleeding in infants, nor is there proof that a caesarean section prevents intracranial bleeding.

10. You can opt not to have the hepatitis B shot given in the hospital, and wait instead. Later, the shot can be given at the pediatrician's office, where you can watch carefully to be sure it's given subcutaneously.

Notes

14 When an Inhibitor Strikes

1. In rare cases, when people who do not have hemophilia are ill, the immune system may malfunction and mistakenly attack factor VIII, creating a condition called acquired hemophilia.

2. Char Witmer and Guy Young, "Factor VIII Inhibitors in Hemophilia A: Rationale and Latest Evidence," *Therapeutic Advances in Hematology* 4.1 (2013): 59–72.

3. Null mutations include large deletions, nonsense mutations, and intron 22 inversions.

4. In contrast, gene mutations such as small deletions or insertions in the DNA coding for factor VIII, which result in the production of a mostly intact factor molecule, result in very low inhibitor rates of about 3%.

5. S. C. Gouw, J. G. van der Bom, and H. Marijke van den Berg, "Treatment-Related Risk Factors of Inhibitor Development in Previously Untreated Patients with Hemophilia A: The CANAL Cohort Study," *Blood* 109 (11): 4648-54.

6. If the test comes back negative, and you still suspect something isn't right, you can request a recovery study, in which factor level measurements are made at 30-minute, 2-hour, 4-hour, 6-hour, and 24-hour intervals after an infusion. A shorter than average half-life can occur without an inhibitor. Treatment can be tailored to stop bleeding in people with a shorter half-life, using more frequent infusions. But without inhibitor testing, there's no way to know if the shorter half-life is normal or due to an inhibitor. Proper treatment can happen only with inhibitor testing first.

7. The test does not directly measure the level of antibodies in the plasma, and results may be affected by other antibodies in the plasma.

8. The Bethesda inhibitor assay is not foolproof. Some people appear to have high-titer inhibitors but respond normally to factor; others have no detectable inhibitors, but infused factor is rapidly neutralized and ineffective.

9. A high-titer inhibitor can reach over 1,000 BU.

10. In some cases, the inhibitor level will drop if the immune system is not exposed to factor for a long time (a year or more). In these cases, standard clotting factor concentrates will often successfully stop a bleed before the immune system ramps up production of the inhibitor that will inactivate the factor.

11. Giuseppe Tagariello, Alfonso Iorio, et al., "High Rate of Spontaneous Inhibitor Clearance during the Long Term Observation Study of a Single Cohort of 524 Haemophilia A Patients Not Undergoing Immunotolerance," *Journal of Hematology and Oncology* 6 (2013): 63.

12. This is called an anamnestic response ("memory response") because it's as if the immune system, which protects your body from germs and viruses, has a memory. The immune system learns to respond more rapidly and powerfully to subsequent exposures to factor than to the first exposure.

13. D. M. DiMichele and B. L. Kroner, "North American Immune Tolerance Study Group. The North American Immune Tolerance Registry: Practices, Outcomes, Outcome Predictors," *Thrombosis and Haemostasis* 87 (2002): 52.

15 Understanding Your Insurance Coverage

1. The information in this chapter represents a general overview only. There are too many variations in healthcare coverage to explain all scenarios in detail. Read this as a starting point to gain insights and increase your awareness of various insurance-related issues.

2. The rising cost of US healthcare has been stunning. In 2013, healthcare spending was $2.9 trillion, or $9,255 per person, representing 17.4% of GDP. The US spends more on healthcare products and services than any other sector. Centers for Medicare and Medicaid Services, http://www.cms.gov/Research-Statistics-Data-and-Systems/Statistics-Trends-and-Reports/NationalHealthExpendData/downloads/highlights.pdf (accessed Nov. 8, 2015).

3. Centers for Disease Control and Prevention, *Report on the Universal Data Collection Program, 2005–2009*, January 2014, 1-26. (accessed Nov. 8, 2015).

4. See Chapter 6 for more on PBMs.

5. A PDL limits approval to use brand name drugs, usually within a therapeutic class. For example, a plan may have a PDL that lists only one brand of recombinant factor VIII. For approval to use a different brand, you may need prior authorization from your physician. A PDL differs slightly from a formulary. For example, the formulary might allow recombinant factor use, but the PDL restricts your choice to one or two brand names of recombinant product.

6. See Chapter 16 for more on patient assistance programs.

7. See Appendix D for sample letters you can write to your insurance company if your coverage for a medically necessary product or service is denied.

16 Maintaining Your Insurance Coverage

1. A.C.C.E.S.S. is a free service funded by PSI that offers in-depth information about public insurance from experienced hemophilia experts.

2. Contact PSI at 800-366-7741.

3. See Appendix B for a list of pharmaceutical company websites.

17 Adolescence and Beyond

1. Testosterone is found in both males and females, but adult males produce about 20 times more testosterone than females.

2. Make it clear to your teen that certain people will always need to know that he has hemophilia, including teachers, coaches, and other parents who shoulder responsibility for him when he travels with them.

3. http://www.drugabuse.gov/publications/drugfacts/high-school-youth-trends (accessed Nov. 8, 2015).

4. NHF's National Youth Leadership Institute (www.hemophilia.org) offers teens and young adults the chance to learn more about personal responsibility, advocacy, and safe networking with others.

5. An amazing number of parents and teens have never heard of statutory rape, or think that marijuana possession is not a serious offense. It pays for you and your teen to know your state laws and the consequences, such as jail sentences.

6. For information on the Selective Service System, see www.sss.gov.

Acknowledgments

For every edition of this book, my first thanks always go to Robert G. Partridge, who in 1989 was a hemophilia product manager at Armour Pharmaceuticals, now CLS Behring LLC. Many people have asked how I, an economist at the time, came to write this book. It's time to tell that tale! One day, while at work, I received Armour's *Hemalog*, a sweet but lightweight family magazine about hemophilia. I wanted to sink my teeth into a real medical and parenting resource, but none existed. The "everything will be okay" message in *Hemalog* left me yearning to know what other parents had experienced. I was desperate to learn what was really in store for my one-year-old, so I could protect him. I tore out the business reply card insert in *Hemalog*, begged for some practical and straightforward info, and dropped it into the mail.

About a week later, *Rob called me at work*. I never dreamed that anyone read these cards, much less acted on them! I apologized to Rob for my critique, but he said that's exactly what he'd wanted. He was listening. He asked, "So what do families with hemophilia need?" I replied, "A Dr. Spock-like book on how to raise a child with hemophilia. I have the first chapter written."

Rob hired me on the spot. And we hadn't even met! Rob had the vision to recognize the need for this book when I proposed it to him in 1989, and he had the business instinct to take a chance on a budding author. He provided funding for this first-of-its-kind book that has changed my life and the lives of thousands of people around the world. Rob and I recently connected on LinkedIn; we enjoyed sharing our memories of those times, and learning what has transpired in our lives since. Without Rob, this book might never have existed, nor any of the books that followed. Thank you, Rob, for completely changing my life and giving me the opportunity to serve an entire community worldwide, and for giving parents the tool they truly need.

I am deeply grateful to the current team at CLS Behring for funding this fifth edition of *Raising a Child with Hemophilia*. CLS Behring, in all its past corporate entities, has been a steady presence and source of support for my publishing on bleeding disorders. The company has also been a donor, helping to fund our projects with the world's poor with hemophilia in developing countries. It has been a joy to collaborate with this inspired team for 25 years. The support we receive from CSL Behring, as well as from other companies, has enabled us to provide all our books and newsletters free of charge to families worldwide for 25 years. Thank you, CSL Behring!

Two people who also have been a steady presence in my life for more than 20 years are my colleagues and good friends Paul Clement and Sara Prisland Evangelos. I could not do the work I do without them; it's as simple as that!

Sara founded JAS Group Writing and Editing, and is the wife of a longtime family friend. She came highly recommended when I realized I needed a medical editor. I can recommend her even more highly now! Sara is the best editor I have ever known and can ever imagine. We have worked together on all of my books and newsletters. Her detailed edits, stirring questions concerning content and meaning, and precise research enrich every aspect of my publications. I am deeply grateful for her commitment to seeking the truth in writing, for questioning my methods and meaning, and for her love of language. When people tell me I am a good writer, I thank them, deflect their praise, and admit, "I have a great editor."

Paul Clement of California, our community's invaluable lay expert on hemophilia, is the father of a child with hemophilia, a retired science teacher, and editor and columnist for the *Parent Empowerment Newsletter (PEN)*. I met Paul and his wife Linda in 1992 at Camp Blood Brothers and Sisters in California, and we have been friends ever since. Paul has the most in-depth knowledge and sharpest research abilities

Acknowledgments

of perhaps anyone in the hemophilia field. He seems to have—or be able to find—the answers to anything, and always presents his results in a fair, unbiased way.

Thank you, Paul and Sara!

My deepest gratitude goes to the over 160 families who have shared their personal stories and advice for all five editions. I'm still in touch with the original 50 families who contacted me, and I've watched their children grow up, go to college, and become parents. It's a joy to be friends on Facebook with people I first read about when they were babies in 1990!

I extend my heartfelt appreciation to the thousands of families with bleeding disorders who have joined our mailing list since 1989. You continue to share your stories with me as we travel on this amazing journey with hemophilia. Thank you all for your faith and trust in me. You've helped me educate others in need. Please continue to share my free resources with new parents who are struggling to find their way.

Finally, in recognition of the role *Hemalog* played in my life, I published the world's first blog dedicated to hemophilia in 2006, and called it *HemaBlog*. I remember my humble roots as a new writer and new parent 25 years ago, but I look forward to the future always. I hope to continue bringing quality information, publications, and humanitarian relief to the worldwide hemophilia community for a long time to come, until the much-prayed-for cure becomes a reality.

APPENDIX A
Publications and Resources

This is a sampling of resources available. Find more by visiting the websites listed here, by searching online, and by contacting NHF and HFA.

BOOKS

Hemophilia
Michelle Raabe
Infobase Publishing 2008
amazon.com
Scientifically detailed, colorful, easy-to-read book focusing on the science behind the treatment, symptoms, genetics of hemophilia. Includes stories of hemophilia's history; how various treatments are made, such as plasma-derived and recombinant; how **gene therapy** might work.

Empower Yourself About Hemophilia
Laureen A. Kelley
LA Kelley Communications, Inc. 2004, 2017
www.kelleycom.com
For families with children newly diagnosed with hemophilia. Includes goal-setting methods and ways to change your perception of hemophilia to help you take charge of your life. Cartoon illustrations of before-and-after situations offer concrete methods to regain control during the rocky first year of hemophilia. Sponsored by Grifols.

Success as a Hemophilia Leader
Laureen A. Kelley
LA Kelley Communications, Inc. 2004, 2017
www.kelleycom.com

World's first guidebook to creating, managing, and growing a grassroots hemophilia organization. Explores creating a vision and mission, forming a board, fundraising, producing a newsletter, programming, establishing an office, and working with a medical advisory board. Offers valuable advice on creating an organization or improving an existing one. Sponsored by Grifols.

Teach Your Child about Hemophilia
Laureen A. Kelley
LA Kelley Communications, Inc. 2007
www.kelleycom.com
www.cslbehring.com
In-depth exploration of the way children understand hemophilia as they mature. Examines children's understanding, at different ages, of hemophilia concepts: cuts, healing, blood, severity levels, blood clotting, infusions, and genetic transmission. Provides a fascinating look at the way children on prophylaxis understand hemophilia. Offers practical tips for answering children's questions. Sponsored by CSL Behring.

A Guide to Living with von Willebrand Disease
Laureen A. Kelley
LA Kelley Communications, Inc. 2017
www.kelleycom.com
www.cslbehring.com
World's first book on the world's most commonly inherited bleeding disorder covers learning to cope with VWD, inheritance, the medical system, treatment, women's issues, and health insurance. Includes a complete resource guide and real-life stories. Sponsored by and available through CSL Behring.

The Gift of Experience: Conversations about Hemophilia
Laura Gray, LICSW, and Christine Chamberlain
Boston Hemophilia Center 2008
Free from NHF
amazon.com
Compilation of personal stories from 21 hemophilia patients born before 1965 and caregivers who treated them. Offers practical information, guidance, support, and insight into caregivers' struggles and achievements.

The Gift of Experience II: Conversations with Parents about Hemophilia
Laura Gray, LICSW, Ziva Mann, and Allie Boutin
Boston Hemophilia Center 2014
Free from NHF
amazon.com
Compilation of personal stories from parents and caregivers of hemophilia patients. Offers insights into the daily life of raising a child with hemophilia.

Dental Care (series)
CSL Behring Consumer Affairs 2010
www.cslbehring.com
Three-part series on dental care, primarily for people and families with hemophilia A, hemophilia B, and VWD. Includes *Dental Care for Infants, Toddlers, and Preschoolers with Bleeding Disorders; Dental Care for Children With Bleeding Disorders: Ages 5 to 10; Dental Care for Adolescents With Bleeding Disorders: Ages 11 to 18.*

A Family Guide to Hemophilia B
CSL Behring 2005
www.mysourcescsl.com
Discusses unique challenges faced by families living with hemophilia B, including treatments and recent advances. Easy-to-understand dosing tools, exercise guides, and self-infusion directions.

Publications on Living with Hemophilia B
Pfizer Inc. 2014
hemophiliavillage.com
Series of ebooks provides insights on living with hemophiia B. Includes *Hemophilia B: A Family Perspective; Hemophilia B in Early Childhood; Navigating the Preteen Years; Hemophilia B: Your Point of View; Young Adults and Hemophilia B; Learn from Experience: A Guide for Mature Adults.*

ELECTRONIC MEDIA

My First Factor Song
Lyrics by Carri Nease
www.kelleycom.com
Sing along and teach through song! To the tune of "Allouette," teach your toddler with hemophilia about bumps, bruises, boo-boos, and factor. Sponsored by Baxalta.

A Bright Future (5-vol. series)
Inalex Communications
www.inalex.com
Series of DVDs includes testimonials from parents on how they coped with the hemophilia diagnosis. Inspires new parents to overcome fear and doubt. Includes *The Hemophilia Diagnosis for Parents; The Hemophilia Diagnosis for the Extended Family; Teaching the Educators; A Time of Transition; Healthy Aging.* Sponsored by Baxalta.

Appendix A

NEWSLETTERS AND MAGAZINES

HemAware
National Hemophilia Foundation
Free with paid NHF membership
www.hemophilia.org
Bimonthly. Newsletter of the largest US hemophilia and bleeding disorder nonprofit. Articles on medical research, treatment, families, and community activities.

Parent Empowerment Newsletter (PEN)
LA Kelley Communications, Inc.
www.kelleycom.com
Quarterly. First US newsletter produced and edited by a parent of a child with hemophilia, and the oldest national newsletter in the bleeding disorder community. Provides medical, scientific, consumer, and parenting articles and news. Empowers parents and patients as educated consumers.

Factor Nine News
Coalition for Hemophilia B
www.coalitionforhemophiliab.org
Quarterly. Newsletter features the latest news and treatment for hemophilia B. From a nonprofit dedicated to improving quality of life for people with hemophilia B by supporting research and education.

Dateline Federation
Hemophilia Federation of America (HFA)
www.hemophiliafed.org
Quarterly. Provides healthcare and advocacy information about bleeding disorders, including upcoming government and healthcare events, innovative programs, and profiles of people with bleeding disorders.

Lifelines
Pfizer Inc.
www.hemophiliavillage.com
Triannual. Newsletter offers information about hemophilia treatment and tips for living an active life, including inspirational stories from people living with hemophilia. Describes latest programs and services available from Pfizer.

Post Script Informer
Patient Services Inc.
www.uneedpsi.org
Quarterly. Newsletter of a nonprofit that specializes in providing temporary insurance coverage to people with chronic medical conditions who face losing insurance. Provides up-to-date information on insurance changes.

FOR CHILDREN

What Is Hemophilia? (series)
Laureen A. Kelley
LA Kelley Communications, Inc. 1995
www.kelleycom.com
English, Spanish
Developmentally arranged series explains hemophilia to children using language and concepts appropriate for three age levels: preschool, school-age, and adolescent. Each book covers the same topics in educationally and cognitively different ways. Contains Note to Parents for each age level

> **Level 1: Joshua, Knight of the Red Snake**
> Empowering story about a preschooler with hemophilia. Illustrated large-text format ends on a note of joy and confidence to empower children. Ages 3–7.

Level 2: They'll Probably Ask You "What is hemophilia?"
Humorous story about Tony, who must explain hemophilia to his fourth-grade classmates. Includes glossary for children. Ages 7–11.

Level 3: Tell Them the Facts!
Question-and-answer book on hemophilia for pre-adolescents and adolescents, and for teachers and parents of newly diagnosed children. Material on genetics is divided into two sections: ages 11–14 and 14–16. Includes glossary.

Must You Always Be a Boy?
Laureen A. Kelley
LA Kelley Communications, Inc. 1991
www.kelleycom.com
Four rhyming tales explore adult reactions to bleeds, overprotective parents, sibling rivalry, and classroom bullies. Illustrated. Ages 3–8.

Alexis: The Prince Who Had Hemophilia
Laureen A. Kelley
LA Kelley Communications, Inc. 1992
www.kelleycom.com
English, Spanish
True story of Alexis, youngest child of Russian Tsar Nicholas II, and how his hemophilia influenced events leading to the Russian revolution. Ages 8 and older.

The Great Inhibinator
Chris Perretti Barnes
BioRX 2006
www.biorx.net
Colorfully illustrated story about Nate, a boy who discovers he has an inhibitor, centers on creating a Halloween costume. Ages 4–7. Sponsored by Bayer HealthCare.

A Drop of Blood
Paul Showers
HarperCollins 2004
Cartoon Halloween characters introduce the basics of blood. Includes why blood is red, blood components, and the role of platelets in blood clotting. Ages 7–11.

My First Factor (series)
Shannon Brush, with illustrations by Brooke Henson
LA Kelley Communications, Inc. 2008-2015
www.kelleycom.com
Series of colorful, chunky books just right for small hands. World's first toddler books for children with hemophilia. Sponsored by Bayer HealthCare. Ages 18 mo.–4 yr.

> **My First Factor Words**
> One-word concepts about family and hemophilia.
>
> **My First Factor: Hemophilia**
> What is hemophilia? Bruises, owie, factor!
>
> **My First Factor: Week**
> Regular infusions help a toddler stay active.
>
> **My First Factor: Fitness**
> Yoga, playing, laughing, and good food keep a toddler healthy.
>
> **My First Factor: HTC**
> Who does a toddler meet at the HTC?
>
> **My First Factor: Infusions**
> A toddler's first look at the steps in an infusion.
>
> **My First Factor: Joints**
> Let's name all our joints! How do they work?

My First Factor: Camp
What will it be like to go to hemophilia camp when you get older?

My First Factor: Self-Infusion
As you grow up, you start doing all kinds of things by yourself!

My First Factor: Safety
How do I stay safe? Ways a child learns to protect himself.

Mis primeras palabras del Factor
A toddler's first book about hemophilia in Spanish.

My First Factor Coloring Book
Illustrations from previous My First Factor books help keep toddlers busy and happy.

Curtis & Jerry on Mount Omega: Adventures with Hemophilia
Celynd Scaglione
BDI Pharma, Inc. 2006
English, Spanish
bookrequest@bdipharma.com
Two young pandas go camping with their fathers and learn what it means to live with hemophilia. Includes information about safe activities for children. Provided by BDI Pharma, Inc.

PROGRAMS

Inalex Communications Workshops for Men
Inalex Communications
www.inalex.com
Workshops and teleconferences for men in the bleeding disorder community offer education and community support. Empowers men to deepen their relationships and deal with anxiety, frustration, stress, anger. Life and executive coaches, social workers, PhD instructors, and bleeding disorder community leaders conduct sessions.

Gettin' in the Game
CSL Behring Consumer Affairs
www.cslbehring.com
Offers local events where children and families can learn sports tips, participate in appropriate exercises and warm-ups, and meet other kids with bleeding disorders.

NHF-CSL Behring Junior National Championship
www.cslbehring.com
Encourages kids with bleeding disorders to be active and stay fit by participating in four baseball and golf regional competitions. Competitions include clinics, art programs, group exercises, and awards.

Dads in Action
Hemophilia Federation of America (HFA)
www.hemophiliafed.org
Network of involved fathers; created to help fathers face the challenges of raising children with bleeding disorders. Provides information, resources, and educational programs.

Helping Hands
Hemophilia Federation of America (HFA)
www.hemophiliafed.org
Offers rapid, noninvasive financial relief for emergency situations. Funds are used to assist qualifying families with housing, transportation, utility, and other one-time emergency needs.

Hope for Hemophilia
www.hopeforhemophilia.com
Nonprofit founded by people with hemophilia that offers financial aid to struggling families with bleeding disorders.

MEDICAL

Patient Notification System (PNS)
Plasma Protein Therapeutics Association (PPTA)
www.patientnotificationsystem.org
Free, confidential, 24-hour communication system provides information on plasma-derived and recombinant product withdrawals and recalls. Offers consumers a single, convenient, confidential source of up-to-date information.

Recommended Websites

CSL Behring
mysourcecsl.com

National Hemophilia Foundation (NHF)
www.hemophilia.org

Hemophilia Federation of America (HFA)
www.hemophiliafed.org

LA Kelley Communications, Inc.
www.kelleycom.com

Coalition for Hemophilia B, Inc.
www.coalitionforhemophiliab.org

Committee of Ten Thousand
www.cott1.org

Centers for Disease Control and Prevention
www.cdc.gov

Hope for Hemophilia
www.hopeforhemophilia.com

Patient Notification System (PNS)
www.patientnotificationsystem.org

Patient Services Inc. (PSI)
www.UneedPSI.org

World Federation of Hemophilia (WFH)
www.wfh.org

Save One Life, Inc.
www.saveonelife.net

APPENDIX B
Pharmaceutical and Medical Device Companies

PHARMACEUTICAL COMPANIES

This is a list of pharmaceutical companies with coagulation and related products licensed in the US and does not represent a product or service endorsement. The list is not necessarily comprehensive.

Akorn Pharmaceuticals
www.akorn.com

Aptevo Therapeutics Inc.
www.aptevotherapeutics.com

AstraZeneca
www.astrazeneca.com

Baxalta
www.baxaltahematology.com

Bayer HealthCare
www.livingwithhemophilia.com

Biogen
www.biogenhemophilia.com

CSL Behring LLC
www.cslbehring-us.com
www.mysourcecsl.com

Ferndale Laboratories, Inc.
www.ferndalelabs.com

Grifols USA
www.grifolsusa.com

Kedrion Biopharma Inc.
www.kedrion.us

Novo Nordisk Inc.
www.novonordisk-us.com

Octapharma USA
www.octapharmausa.com

Pfizer Inc.
www.hemophiliavillage.com

Shire
www.shire.com

Teva Pharmaceuticals
www.tevausa.com

MEDICAL DEVICE COMPANIES

MedicAlert Foundation
www.medicalert.org
Products: MedicAlert® identification cards and jewelry

APPENDIX C
Sample Letters

A. Sample Emergency Care Letter

This letter should be typed on your doctor's letterhead and signed by your doctor.

Date: 8/12/15

PATIENT INFORMATION

Name: Johnny Doe	Date of birth: 2/15/2005
Address: 1234 Any Street, Anytown, State 12345	Phone: (123) 123-1233
Emergency contact: Mary Doe	Home phone: (123) 123-1234
Relationship to patient: Mother	Cell: (123) 123-1235
Hematologist name: Dr. Clott	
Doctor phone: (123) 456-4567	Doctor fax: (123) 456-4568
Doctor cell: (123) 456-4569	Doctor signature:_____

DIAGNOSIS AND TREATMENT INFORMATION

Diagnosis: Severe factor VIII deficiency (hemophilia A)

Synopsis: Hemophilia A is an inherited bleeding disorder caused by a deficiency of factor VIII (FVIII). Signs and symptoms include severe bruising, spontaneous bleeding into joints or muscles, and prolonged bleeding following injury, surgery, and dental work.

Drug allergies: PCN, ASA

Patient weight: 32 kg

Routine medications: None

Recommended treatment for bleeding episodes: Bleeding in patients with severe hemophilia requires infusions of **antihemophilic factor** (factor VIII concentrate).

- Minor hemorrhage (superficial, early hemorrhages, hemorrhages into joints): 10–20 IU FVIII per kg. Repeat dose if evidence of further bleeding.
- Moderate to major hemorrhage (hemorrhages into muscles or oral cavity; hemarthroses; known trauma); surgery (minor surgical procedures): 15–30 IU FVIII per kg. Repeat one dose at 12–24 hours if needed.
- Major to life-threatening hemorrhage (intracranial, intra-abdominal, intra-thoracic hemorrhages; gastrointestinal or central nervous system bleeding; bleeding in retropharyngeal or retroperitoneal spaces or iliopsoas compartment); fractures

and head trauma: Initial dose 40–50 IU FVIII per kg. Repeat dose 20–25 IU FVIII per kg every 8–12 hours.
- Surgery (major surgical procedures): Preoperative dose 50 IU FVIII per kg. Verify 100% activity prior to surgery. Repeat as necessary after 6–12 hours initially, and for 10–14 days until healing is complete.
- Mouth and mucous membrane bleeding: Antifibrinolytic agent (Amicar) in conjunction with factor concentrate.

PRECAUTIONS

Procedural precautions: Patient must be pretreated with factor concentrate prior to diagnostic tests, surgery or invasive procedures such as NG tube insertion, chest tube insertion, or LP. Use less invasive procedures whenever possible. Avoid nasal intubation. Routine venipunctures do not require pretreatment. Routine **coagulation** testing such as PT/PTT/BT does not assist with the management of hemophilia. Avoid IM injections; SQ are preferred.

Medication precautions: Avoid aspirin and most NSAIDs because they interfere with platelet function. Celebrex, Trilisate, and Disalcid (salsalate) are acceptable. Opiates are safe, but avoid ASA combinations; use acetaminophen/Tylenol combinations instead.

B. Sample Appeal Letter to Insurance Company for Denial of Coverage #1

For denial of brand of factor concentrate. Can be adapted for other accepted standard-of-care treatments such as denials for Amicar or for hepatitis immunization.

VIA CERTIFIED MAIL, RETURN RECEIPT REQUESTED

Dr. B. N. Denial
Medical Director
Major US Insurance, Inc.
1234 Any Street
Any Town, Any State 12345
RE: Denial of Coverage for Factor Brand
Member number: 3TTXYZ
Date: Aug. 12, 2015

Appendix C

Dear Dr. Denial,

My 10-year-old son, John, has severe factor VIII deficiency (hemophilia A). Hemophilia is an inherited blood disorder that causes prolonged bleeding. This bleeding occurs mainly in joints, but can occur anywhere in the body. Bleeding in the joints damages cartilage and can lead to permanent crippling.

Treatment for my son involves intravenous infusions of factor VIII concentrate, which contains the clotting protein that his blood lacks. The brand prescribed by my son's hematologist is [*factor concentrate name*]. Recently I tried to obtain this factor concentrate for use at home. Your company denied coverage. Your company stated that this brand of factor concentrate was too expensive, that it was not in the formulary, and that a different brand should be administered.

Perhaps the initial denial was due to lack of adequate information about hemophilia treatment. Please immediately authorize coverage of this brand of factor concentrate for use in home therapy. The standard of care in the bleeding disorder community promotes home use of all brands of factor concentrate, either self-administered or administered by a trained family member or home care nurse. Not all brands of factor are equal. My policy with your company clearly states that the plan will pay for all medically necessary services and products as prescribed by a physician.

By refusing to authorize this medically necessary and FDA-approved therapy for purely financial reasons, your company is denying my son the nationally accepted standard of care for his disorder.

Thank you for reconsidering this denial of coverage and for any assistance you can provide. I await your prompt reply.

Very truly yours,
Your name
Address
Phone
Policy number
Enclosure
Cc: Your lawyer
Your home care company representative
Your hematologist

C. Sample Appeal Letter to Insurance Company For Denial of Coverage #2

For denial of home therapy. Can be adapted for denial of other accepted standard-of-care treatments.

VIA CERTIFIED MAIL, RETURN RECEIPT REQUESTED

Mrs. I.M. Controller
Claims Administrator
Major US Insurance, Inc.
1234 Any Street
Any Town, Any State 12345
RE: Denial of Coverage for Home Therapy
Member number: 3TTXYZ
Date: Aug. 12, 2015

Dear Ms. Controller,

Two weeks ago, I was informed by [factor provider] that you have denied payment for home use of [factor concentrate name], a blood clotting medicine my son uses to treat bleeding resulting from his hemophilia. He first began using [factor concentrate name] in March 2006. Prior to home use in 2008, we had to go to his HTC clinic, or local emergency room, for infusions to treat his bleeding episodes. This was far more costly and time-consuming than home infusions, which we are now trained to do.

Your company has been reimbursing [factor provider] for [factor concentrate name] for 26 months. Suddenly, and with no adequate explanation, you denied the most recent order. My insurance policy with your company clearly states that the plan will pay for those services and medications determined medically necessary and prescribed by a physician. Enclosed you will find a letter from my son's hematologist outlining my son's condition and his continued need for home therapy. Unless your company's denial was based on a review of son's case by a board-certified hematologist who specializes in the management of hemophilia, you have breached your contract with me.

I request an immediate review of this denial. In the interim, my son's supplies of [factor concentrate name] are running low, and we will need to return to the HTC clinic or ER for every bleeding episode. This will add thousands of dollars to your reimbursement, and will put my son's short-term and long-term health at risk because

Appendix C

he will continue to bleed as we transport him and wait at these medical centers for treatment. I await your prompt reply.

Very truly yours,
Your name
Address
Phone
Policy number
Enclosure
Cc: Your lawyer
Your home care company representative
Your hematologist

APPENDIX D
History and Significance of Blood Product Safety

Paul Clement

Clotting factor concentrates used to treat bleeding in people with hemophilia are classified as either recombinant or plasma-derived. These two classifications refer to the origin of the product. Recombinant products are made in the laboratory, typically from animal cells containing human genes but not from human blood. Plasma-derived products come from human blood, or more specifically, plasma, the liquid portion of the blood.

Any pharmaceutical product manufactured using human blood or blood plasma can potentially transmit blood-borne illnesses, such as viral infections. Before the mid 1980s, factor concentrates were not virally inactivated, meaning that viruses in the plasma used to make the factor could survive the manufacturing process and still be infectious. As a result, people with hemophilia—and anyone using a blood product—could potentially contract any viral disease that happened to be in the nation's blood supply. Although some viruses, such as **hepatitis C** (HCV), were known to be in the blood supply, some new or "emerging" viruses, such as the human immunodeficiency virus (HIV), were unknown.[1]

Today's plasma-derived factor concentrates are considerably safer than those of the past. Improved donor screening methods, better purification methods capable of removing viruses, and effective viral inactivation procedures have drastically reduced the risk of viral transmission. Most recombinant products also undergo viral inactivation procedures, but because they are not made from blood, the risk of viral transmission is hypothetical. Although we've made progress, the bleeding disorder community continues to monitor the safety of plasma-derived factor concentrates. Why? Because the integrity of the blood supply is constantly challenged by emerging viruses. To understand how plasma-derived factor concentrate is kept safe, you need to to understand how it's made.

Donor Screening

Plasma-derived factor concentrate is made from the pooled plasma of tens of thousands of donors. Donors are recruited from people considered at low risk of having viral infections.[2]

Before their first donation, potential blood or plasma donors are screened through rigorous interviews. They're asked if they practice any high-risk behaviors, such as using intravenous (IV) drugs or having multiple sexual partners. A "yes" answer excludes them as donors: they are "deferred" from donating their plasma or blood. Plasmapheresis centers—locations where plasma donations are made—also often require donors to have a medical exam. Unsuitable donors are entered into a national registry, called the *donor deferral list*, to prevent the use of their plasma nationwide.

Blood or plasma donations from people who have passed the initial screening process are then carefully tested for viral markers, to detect the presence of viruses that cause infectious diseases such as hepatitis and HIV. Plasma from a donor who tests positive for an infectious virus is destroyed, and the donor is rejected and placed on the donor deferral list.

If a donor tests negative, that person's donated plasma is then frozen and quarantined for 60 days[3] until the donor donates a second time and passes the viral testing again. This extra step protects against possible infection during the *window period*. The window period is the length of time it takes, after infection by a virus such as HIV, for the virus to become detectable by diagnostic tests. During the window period, a person infected with HIV or another virus will not show up on diagnostic tests as being infected, even though he or she is infectious.

The window period varies from virus to virus, and also varies with the type of diagnostic test being used. To test for HIV, there are three basic types of diagnostic tests: (1) antibody tests, (2) **antigen** tests, and (3) nucleic acid tests.

Antibody tests don't look for the virus itself, but instead test for the presence of antibodies, produced by the immune system, that target HIV. HIV tests are often called first-, second-, third- or fourth-generation tests. First- and second-generation antibody tests detect only one type of antibody against HIV. On average, they can detect antibodies 42 to 60 days after infection (meaning these tests have a window period of 42–60 days). Third-generation antibody tests can detect all types of antibodies, and can detect antibodies in about 21 to 24 days.

Antigen tests check for the presence of a specific protein from the virus (such as the p24 antigen from HIV) that appears in the blood before antibodies are produced by the immune system. Tests for the p24 antigen can detect HIV within about 10 days of infection. The p24 antigen test is not used by itself because, although the antigen level is high at the beginning of the infection, it drops off to undetectable levels after the HIV infection becomes fully established; for this reason, the test may give a false negative result. Fourth-generation HIV tests are a combination of antibody and antigen tests: the antigen portion of the test picks up the early-stage infection p24 antigen, and the antibody portion of the test picks up the presence of antibodies that occur later, after the body responds to the infection.

Nucleic acid tests (NAT) detect genetic material from the virus itself, and don't rely on the presence of antibodies or antigens.[4] There are several types of NAT, but a common type is the polymerase chain reaction (PCR) test. NAT can detect HIV about 12 days after infection.

NAT is routinely used to test for HIV in donated pools of blood or plasma, but because it's expensive, it's not routinely used to test for HIV in individuals. NAT is used to test for HIV in babies born to HIV-positive mothers because babies retain the mother's antibodies for several months after birth, making the antibody test inaccurate. NAT is used by factor manufacturers to test small pools of plasma for the presence of several viruses—including hepatitis A and B viruses (HAV and HBV), HCV, HIV, and human **parvovirus B19** (HPV B19)—before the plasma is combined into large pools for processing. NAT can significantly shorten the window period by detecting the genetic material of infectious viruses much earlier than antibody tests.

After passing all the viral screening tests, the plasma is frozen and shipped to the manufacturing plant, where it's thawed and combined with the plasma of tens of thousands of other donors to be *fractionated*. **Fractionation** is the process that separates the plasma into different parts, including clotting factors. The fractionated parts are then purified, undergo procedures to inactivate or filter out viruses, and are packaged as the final product.

Purification and Viral Inactivation

The fractionation and purification processes used to make plasma-derived factor concentrates also remove most of the viruses in the factor, but they don't completely eliminate the risk of viral infection. To eliminate or greatly reduce the chance of viral infection, the production process must include (1) a filtration process and/or (2) a viral inactivation process.

All plasma-derived factor concentrates are purified to remove most unwanted proteins and reduce the number of viruses. But some factor concentrates undergo an additional purification step that can remove almost all viruses. Passing clotting factor through filters with very small pores, a process called *nanofiltration*, can effectively remove viruses based on their size: the viruses are stopped by the filter because they're too large to pass through.

The two main viral inactivation methods are (1) heat treatment, such as pasteurization, and (2) washing with chemicals, known as solvent-detergent washing.[5] These viral inactivation methods can inactivate HIV, hepatitis B (HBV), and hepatitis C (HCV), but they can't inactivate all viruses.

Why can't all viruses be inactivated? Viruses can be divided into two groups: **lipid-enveloped** and **non-enveloped**. Viral inactivation processes do not affect the two groups of viruses in the same way.

Lipid-enveloped viruses have a fatty coating; they include HIV, HBV, and HCV. They are susceptible to heat and solvent-detergent viral inactivation processes.

Non-enveloped viruses don't have a fatty coating, or lipid envelope; they include HAV and HPV B19. Heat and solvent-detergent viral inactivation processes are not effective against non-enveloped viruses. And these processes have no effect on the agents that cause Creutzfeldt-Jakob disease (CJD). But recent laboratory studies have found that purification processes used to manufacture plasma products are capable of removing most CJD agents.

What Viruses or Diseases Are of Greatest Concern?

Infectious diseases are commonly caused by bacteria, protozoans (one-celled organisms, such as those that cause malaria and giardia), and viruses. Fortunately, bacteria and protozoans are easily killed or inactivated by the fractionation and production processes used to make plasma-derived clotting factor. Assuming there is no breach in the quality control procedures of the manufacturing process, no blood diseases caused by bacteria or protozoans can be transmitted by clotting factor.

By contrast, viruses are much harder to destroy or remove from plasma. It's fortunate that the viruses responsible for serious diseases such as HIV and two of the three types of hepatitis are lipid-enveloped. These viruses have a fatty outer layer and are easily inactivated by heat and solvent-detergent viral inactivation processes. But some viruses and agents of disease, such as those that cause CJD, are difficult or impossible to inactivate with current viral inactivation methods:

Hepatitis A virus. HAV is usually not a blood-borne disease. It normally spreads when people drink water, eat food, or touch objects contaminated by fecal matter from an HAV-infected person. It also spreads through intimate contact with the saliva of an infected person (kissing someone with HAV or having sexual contact). Anyone is at risk. HAV may be passed quickly in daycare centers and other settings with inadequate hand washing. Infection with HAV usually results in a short-term illness. Symptoms include runny nose, diarrhea, and a fever over 100 °F. An adolescent with HAV may have jaundice (yellowing of the skin), dark urine, or pain in the liver (right abdominal area). Adults tend to get sicker than children.

Symptoms usually clear up in about a month, although some people who can't clear the virus develop chronic hepatitis (liver inflammation). A person with HCV or HBV who also gets HAV will have a more severe, potentially fatal illness. There is no known treatment, but a vaccine is available to prevent HAV. People with bleeding disorders who use blood products should be vaccinated against HAV and also HBV.[6]

Human parvovirus B19. Discovered in 1974, HPV B19 causes a common childhood disorder known as fifth disease or erythema infectiosum. Symptoms include fever, rash, joint pain, and a general feeling of discomfort. The virus usually lasts about a week, and full recovery is the norm. Most adults who were exposed to HPV B19 during childhood, and have built up immunity to it, will not become clinically ill if infected again. HPV B19 may cause fetal complications in women who become infected during pregnancy. In the general population, 30% to 60% of adults have antibodies against HPV B19, indicating a past infection. However, more than 90% of people with hemophilia have antibodies to HPV B19, and the more plasma-derived clotting factor they receive, the more likely they are to have antibodies to HPV B19—this relationship indicates that people who use clotting factor are being exposed to HPV B19 through the factor.

Like HAV, HPV B19 is a non-enveloped virus and has been detected in both solvent-detergent and heat-treated factor concentrate. It's also one of the smallest viruses, so it's hard to remove by filtration. Some manufacturers are now using PCR testing to screen source plasma (plasma collected through a process called plasmapheresis) for HPV B19, and are working on ways to remove it from factor concentrate.

Creutzfeldt-Jakob disease. CJD is a rare neurological disease that belongs to a class of diseases called *transmissible* spongiform encephalopathies (TSEs). These diseases are transmissible, meaning they can be transmitted to others under certain conditions. An *encephalopathy* is a disease of the brain; and *spongiform* refers to the "spongy" appearance of the brain caused by TSEs. TSEs are untreatable and always fatal. One extremely rare form of CJD is inherited. In some cases, CJD has been transmitted by medical procedures, such as the implantation of dura mater (a graft of the covering of the brain) or cornea from the cadavers of infected people; or through the use of human growth hormone derived from cadavers of infected people. Some infections have occurred after eating meat from animals with TSEs (see next section, variant CJD). But the majority of cases are of unknown origin and are called *sporadic CJD*.

Appendix D

CJD is not caused by a virus but by a *CJD prion*, a variant of a normally occurring human prion protein. Prions are found mostly in nerve tissue and are especially abundant in the brain. The exact function of normal prions is unknown. CJD prions are misfolded forms of normal human prion proteins. Prions are not living, and do not multiply like viruses or bacteria, but they're able to start a chain reaction by converting the normal prions into misfolded, water-insoluble CJD prions. Because the body is unable to remove these misfolded CJD prions, they accumulate in brain tissue, eventually killing nerves, and leading to progressively degenerative and invariably fatal neurological diseases.

The accumulation of CJD prions can happen over decades before symptoms are visible, and the disease is not easily diagnosed. Currently, no commercially available blood test exists to detect CJD. The only way to positively diagnose CJD is by examining the brain after the patient has died. But this may change in the near future: in 2014, researchers in the United Kingdom reported some success in developing a blood test to detect a form of CJD called *variant CJD* (vCJD). And further studies on this blood test may prove that it can detect CJD; this could lead to a commercial blood test for vCJD.

Variant Creutzfeldt-Jakob disease. vCJD is a TSE caused by eating beef from cows who have a CJD-like disease called bovine spongiform encephalopathy (BSE), also known as mad cow disease. BSE is a neurological disease of cows that is also caused by CJD prions and, in rare cases, can be transmitted to people who eat BSE-contaminated meat.

CJD prions have been found in blood and other tissues of infected patients. Although four people contracted vCJD after receiving vCJD-contaminated blood transfusions between December 2003 and April 2007, no cases have been reported of CJD or vCJD transmission through fractionated blood products such as clotting factor. Based on the few cases of CJD transmitted through blood, it appears that neither CJD nor vCJD is easily transmitted through blood. The risk of CJD transmission through plasma-derived factor is considered extremely small, because the fractionation process and purification processes used to make factor are capable of removing most, if not all, prions from the final product.

Still, CJD is not a nationally reportable disease in the United States, meaning we don't know the actual number of CJD cases. And CJD is often misdiagnosed as Alzheimer's or other neurological disorders. Because we also lack a blood test, and because of CJD's long incubation period, it's currently impossible to get an accurate risk assessment. As a precaution, in November 1999, regulatory authorities including the FDA recommended the withdrawal of all plasma-derived products made from the plasma of anyone who is later diagnosed with vCJD. The authorities also recommended that blood donors be deferred based on their potential exposure to BSE in the UK (e.g., eating beef) or their use of bovine (cow) insulin made in the UK.

Why We Need to Watchdog Our Factor and Blood Supply

Donor screening procedures and viral inactivation methods help keep products safe. Another safety measure is the tracking of products *after* they reach the market. Unwanted side effects, known as *adverse events*, experienced as a result of using a factor concentrate are monitored regularly to detect problems with the product or production process. Consumers may report adverse events directly to the FDA. But more likely, a patient will report an adverse event to a physician, who then forwards the information to the FDA and factor manufacturer. Manufacturers are required to report adverse events related to the product to the FDA. Adverse events may include anaphylaxis resulting when someone with factor IX inhibitors infuses a factor IX concentrate; or the development of

Appendix D

inhibitors. Reporting adverse events helps identify potential problems with the product or manufacturing process.

Despite continuing efforts to improve blood safety, *no blood product is guaranteed 100% safe*. Blood safety involves developing and implementing effective prevention strategies to minimize the risk of potential blood-borne infections. Safety requires vigilant surveillance of the blood supply for known and emerging agents of disease. New treatments or vaccines can eliminate the risks of some viruses. But emerging viruses may pose new threats. There is always a risk associated with using a plasma-derived product or a product that contains plasma proteins such as albumin. All parents and patients need to stay up-to-date on new developments in blood safety by reading literature and news briefs from NHF, HFA, COTT, your HTC and local hemophilia organizations, manufacturers, and home care companies.

---

1. An emerging virus is one that has adapted to cause an infectious disease. Emerging viruses either were never known, or were known in animal or human populations without causing a disease, but then mutated to cause disease.

2. This is in contrast to how plasma was collected decades ago, when donations were sought from prisoners and people living in the "skid row" areas of cities who were at high risk of carrying viral diseases.

3. In 1997, Plasma Protein Therapeutics Association (PPTA) implemented the Quality, Safety, Excellence, Assurance and Leadership (QSEAL) certification program for plasma manufacturers. This program and its associated standards are voluntary and go beyond what's required by law. NHF's MASAC endorses the QSEAL certification program and standards as important ways to ensure that only the highest-quality plasma is collected and used for manufacturing plasma-derived factor.

4. Antigens are proteins on the surface of a virus that elicit an immune response.

5. Additional viral inactivation methods are currently under investigation.

6. In the US bleeding disorder community, HAV made headlines in the mid-1990s when four people contracted HAV from factor concentrates. It was found that several batches of plasma-derived factor concentrate were made from a plasma pool that tested positive for HAV. The affected factor used a solvent-detergent viral inactivation method. HAV is not a lipid-enveloped virus, so it is not susceptible to the solvent-detergent process. HAV is also relatively resistant to heat treatments such as pasteurization. However, transmission of HAV has never been confirmed in a pasteurized plasma-derived product.

APPENDIX E
Medicines to Avoid

This list does not contain all the products available that should be avoided or used only with caution and medical advice. Get medical advice before taking any prescription product, or any non-prescription product that might interact with treatment for your condition.

Products Containing Aspirin

Please note that this is an incomplete list. Dozens of drugs contain *aspirin*. The word aspirin may not appear on the drug label. Some medication labels may use terms such as ASA, acetylsalicylate, acetylsalicylic acid, salicylic, salicylamide, or phenyl salicylate instead of the word *aspirin*.

- acetylsalicylic acid (ASA)†
- Alka-Seltzer®
- Anacin®
- Anexsia® (hydrocodone bitartrate and acetaminophen)
- APC‡
- Ascriptin®
- Bufferin®
- Darvon® with ASA (propoxyphene hydrochloride and aspirin)
- Darvon® Compound-65 (propoxyphene hydrochloride, aspirin and caffeine capsules, USP)
- Dristan®
- Ecotrin®
- Empirin® with Codeine (aspirin and codeine phosphate)
- Equagesic® (meprobamate with aspirin)
- Excedrin®
- Fiorinal® (butalbital, aspirin, caffeine)
- Lortab® with aspirin (hydrocodone bitartrate, aspirin); Lortab without aspirin is safe to take.
- P-A-C® Compound

†Generic name for aspirin. ‡Abbreviation for aspirin, phenacetin, and caffeine.

Pepto-Bismol®
Percodan® (oxycodone hydrochloride, oxycodone terephthalate, aspirin, USP)
Percodan®-Demi (oxycodone hydrochloride and aspirin)
Robaxisal® (methocarbamol, USP/aspirin, USP)
Synalgos®-DC
Vanquish®
Zorprin®

Nonsteroidal Anti-inflammatory Drugs (NSAIDs)

Use with medical advice.

Advil®
Aleve®
Arthrotec® (diclofenac sodium/misoprostol)
Cataflam® (diclofenac potassium)
Clinoril® (sulindac)
Daypro®
Dolobid® (diflunisal)
Feldene® (piroxicam)
ibuprofen§
Indocin®
indomethacin§
Lodine® (etodolac)
Motrin®
Naprelan®
Naprosyn®
naproxen§
Nuprin®
Orudis®
Ponstel® (mefenamic acid)
Tolectin® (tolmetin sodium)
Toradol® (ketorolac tromethamine)
Vicoprofen®
Voltaren® (diclofenac sodium)

§Generic name for one of the NSAIDs.

APPENDIX F
Factor VIII Dosage Calculation Chart

Factor VIII units to be administered *

Patient's Weight	Desired Increase in Circulating Factor (%)							
	30%	40%	50%	60%	70%	80%	90%	100%
10 lbs./4.5 kg	68	90	113	135	158	180	203	225
11 lbs./4.9 kg	74	98	123	147	172	196	221	245
12 lbs./5.4 kg	81	108	135	162	189	216	243	270
13 lbs./5.8 kg	87	116	145	174	203	232	261	290
14 lbs./6.3 kg	95	126	158	189	221	252	284	315
15 lbs./6.7 kg	101	134	168	201	235	268	302	335
16 lbs./7.2 kg	108	144	180	216	252	288	324	360
17 lbs./7.6 kg	114	152	190	228	266	304	342	380
18 lbs./8.1 kg	122	162	203	243	284	324	365	405
19 lbs./8.5 kg	128	170	213	255	298	340	383	425
20 lbs./9.0 kg	135	180	225	270	315	360	405	450
31 lbs./14 kg	210	280	350	420	490	560	630	700
40 lbs./18 kg	270	360	450	540	630	720	810	900
51 lbs./23 kg	345	460	575	690	805	920	1035	1150
59 lbs./27 kg	405	540	675	810	945	1080	1215	1350
70 lbs./32 kg	480	640	800	960	1120	1280	1440	1600
79 lbs./36 kg	540	720	900	1080	1260	1440	1620	1800
90 lbs./41 kg	615	820	1025	1230	1435	1640	1845	2050
99 lbs./45 kg	675	900	1125	1350	1575	1800	2025	2250
110 lbs./50 kg	750	1000	1250	1500	1750	2000	2250	2500
121 lbs./55 kg	825	1100	1375	1650	1925	2200	2475	2750
130 lbs./59 kg	885	1180	1475	1770	2065	2360	2655	2950
141 lbs./64 kg	960	1280	1600	1920	2240	2560	2880	3200
150 lbs./68 kg	1020	1360	1700	2040	2380	2720	3060	3400
161 lbs./73 kg	1095	1460	1825	2190	2555	2920	3285	3650
169 lbs./77 kg	1155	1540	1925	2310	2695	3080	3465	3850
180 lbs./82 kg	1230	1640	2050	2460	2870	3280	3690	4100
189 lbs./86 kg	1290	1720	2150	2580	3010	3440	3870	4300
200 lbs./91 kg	1365	1820	2275	2730	3185	3640	4095	4550

Appendix F

Directions for Use

1. Locate patient weight.
2. Choose desired increase in factor VIII.
3. Note factor VIII units to be administered and reconstitute accordingly.
4. Or use this formula: weight (lbs) ÷ 4.4 × factor level desired = number of factor VIII units needed.
5. For factor IX dosage, double all of the numbers of units in chart.

Note: Correct dosage depends on your child's weight and the severity of the bleed (see Chapter 3). *For severe bleeds, always contact your child's hematologist for proper dosing of factor.*

* All fractional values have been rounded to the nearest whole unit. Factor is not available in exact doses. It is sold in about a half-dozen potency ranges, also known as assays, starting from about 250 IU per vial up to about 4,000 IU per vial. The exact number of units per vial often varies per lot. The pharmacy will typically order factor with a potency that is closest to the number of units of factor prescribed by your physician, usually within 10% of the prescribed dose. If factor potencies available at the time of the pharmacy order are not within 10% of the prescribed dose, it is always better to infuse more factor (higher potency) rather than less factor (lower potency). Always infuse the entire contents of the factor vial. Some pharmacies may provide you with several lots of factor of differing potencies and ask you to combine three to six or more vials to make one dose. This practice is unacceptable. Preferably, ask your pharmacy to provide you with one or, at most, two potencies to make one dose.

APPENDIX G
Product Trademarks

Current as of July 1, 2016

Amicar®

Broviac®

Cheerios®

DDAVP®

EMLA®

EpiPen®

Gomco Clamp

Hickman®

L.M.X.4®

MedicAlert®

Plastibell®

Popsicles®

Tegaderm™

Terumo BCT winged infusion set

Tylenol®

Glossary

Most of the terms in this glossary are defined as they relate to hemophilia.

Acetaminophen: Analgesic (pain medication) used to reduce pain and fever.

Acquired hemophilia: Rare autoimmune disorder in which the immune system mistakenly attacks factor VIII. Often triggered by illness; usually occurs in the elderly. Symptoms include extensive soft tissue and internal bleeds, but rarely joint bleeds. Males and females are both affected.

Acquired immune deficiency syndrome (AIDS): Advanced stage in the breakdown of the immune system resulting from infection with the human immunodeficiency virus (HIV). As damage to the immune system progresses, the body becomes increasingly vulnerable to opportunistic life-threatening infections and cancers not normally seen in someone with a properly functioning immune system.

Activated prothrombin complex concentrate (aPCC): Special factor concentrate used to stop bleeding in patients with inhibitors.

Advocate: 1. To speak or write in favor of, as in standing up for oneself or another or defending a position; having input to support one's opinion. 2. One who represents, stands up for, or defends another.

Affordable Care Act (ACA): Two separate pieces of legislation—the Patient Protection and Affordable Care Act (P.L. 111-148) and the Health Care and Education Reconciliation Act of 2010 (P.L. 111-152)—that together implemented a series of comprehensive health insurance reforms, including the expansion of Medicaid coverage to millions of low-income Americans.

AIDS: SEE ACQUIRED IMMUNE DEFICIENCY SYNDROME.

Albumin (or human serum albumin): Protein found in blood plasma that makes up about 50% of plasma proteins. In some brands of recombinant factor concentrate, albumin is added to the final product as a stabilizer or used in the production process.

Amicar (aminocaproic acid): Brand name of an antifibrinolytic drug that prevents enzymes from dissolving clots. Useful in helping to retain clots on mucous membrane bleeds, as in the mouth, nose, and intestines. SEE ANTIFIBRINOLYTIC.

Amniocentesis (or amniotic fluid test, AFT): Prenatal diagnostic test, performed between weeks 13 and 16 of gestation, used to detect certain chromosomal abnormalities and identify the sex of the fetus. Can accurately diagnose hemophilia.

Analgesic: Painkiller or pain medication.

Anamnestic response: Activation of the immune system's memory of foreign substances it has previously encountered, triggering the rapid formation of antibodies when the same foreign substance is encountered again. In inhibitor patients, the anamnestic response causes a fast rise in the inhibitor titer (BU) after exposure to factor. SEE BETHESDA UNIT.

Anaphylaxis: Severe, potentially life-threatening whole-body allergic reaction, sometimes occurring after a factor infusion. Although anaphylaxis is rare, people with hemophilia B and inhibitors are at significantly higher risk if infused with factor IX.

Ancillaries: Medical supplies used during an infusion. May include syringe, needles, medical tape, adhesives, alcohol swabs, gauze.

Anemia: Most common blood condition, caused by a low red blood cell count and resulting in fatigue and weakness. May be caused by an iron-deficient diet, bleeding, or some hepatitis C drugs.

Antibodies: Blood proteins produced by the immune system in response to foreign substances, such as bacteria or viruses, in the bloodstream. Antibodies are programmed to identify, cling to, inactivate, and mark foreign substances for destruction and removal. Antibodies are created to attack a certain virus or protein, and no other.

Antifibrinolytic: Class of drugs that slow fibrinolysis, the breakdown of blood clots. SEE AMICAR.

Antigen: Any substance that causes the immune system to produce antibodies.

Antihemophilic factor (AHF): Another name for commercially produced factor VIII.

Arteries: Largest blood vessels. Arteries bring oxygenated blood from the lungs to the rest of the body.

Arthropathy: Disease of a joint. SEE HEMOPHILIC ARTHROPATHY.

Aseptic: Processes or techniques designed to minimize contamination with microorganisms.

Aspirin (acetylsalicylic acid, ASA): Analgesic. Should never be used by people with blood-clotting disorders because it interferes with the formation of a clot. SEE ANALGESIC.

Assay: Laboratory test that measures the amount or activity of a drug or biochemical substance.

Bethesda unit (BU): Measure of an inhibitor level (titer). Indicates the ability of the inhibitor to neutralize factor, preventing it from helping to form a blood clot. Expressed as a number: the higher the BU, the more powerful the inhibitor and the less effective a factor infusion will be. BU measurements vary from less than 1 to over 9,000. BU measurements over 5 inactivate almost all infused factor, often within minutes, and require bypassing agents to control bleeds. SEE TITER, BYPASSING AGENT.

Breakthrough bleeds: Spontaneous bleeds that occur while a person is on prophylaxis.

Butterfly needle: Needle with "wings" (tabs) on either side used for venipuncture, allowing precise placement of the needle in a vein. On one end of the needle is narrow, flexible tubing with a connector for attachment to a syringe or other device.

Bypassing agent: Blood-clotting product that skips the steps in the clotting process where factor VIII or IX is needed. Useful for inhibitor patients, who often can't use regular factor VIII or IX products.

Cap: Maximum limit of reimbursable medical expenses allowed by an insurance policy.

Capillaries: Tiniest blood vessels. Capillaries bring oxygenated blood from arteries to tissues of the body.

Carrier: Person who has a gene for a certain trait, but who does not normally exhibit that trait.

Carrier test: One of several blood tests that can determine whether a female has the hemophilia gene. When she knows her carrier status, she can make more informed family planning decisions.

Cauterization: Process of burning with a hot needle, laser, or electrical current for medical reasons, for example, to seal off a bleeding blood vessel.

Central venous access device (CVAD): Medical device used for IV infusions without having to access a vein. CVADs include internal devices, called ports, and external devices, also called central lines.

Chorionic villus sampling (CVS): Prenatal test used to diagnosis hemophilia that samples tissue from the placenta, either through a long, thin needle inserted into the abdomen or through a thin, flexible tube inserted through the cervix. Testing shows the presence or absence of hemophilia genetic markers. Performed between weeks 10 and 12 of pregnancy, with an accuracy rate above 99%.

Glossary

Christmas disease: Another name for hemophilia B or factor IX deficiency. Named in 1952 after Stephen Christmas, the first patient to be diagnosed with factor IX deficiency.

Chromatography: Any of many different processes used to separate a complex mixture into its parts. In producing factor concentrates, chromatography is used to separate factor VIII or IX from other blood proteins to increase the purity of the factor. **Monoclonal antibody purification,** often used to purify factor concentrates, is a type of chromatography. SEE MONOCLONAL ANTIBODY PURIFICATION.

Chromosome: Structure that contains the genes within the nucleus of each cell.

Circumcision: Surgical removal of the foreskin of the penis. Excessive bleeding resulting from this elective surgery is a common way that families with no known history of hemophilia discover their child has hemophilia.

Clotting cascade: Series of cellular and chemical reactions involving the 13 blood-clotting factors in response to an injured blood vessel. Ends with the formation of fibrin fibers in the platelet plug, forming a blood clot.

Clotting factor: SEE FACTOR, FACTOR CONCENTRATE.

Coagulation: Formation of a blood clot.

COBRA: Consolidated Omnibus Budget Reconciliation Act of 1985. Allows patients to temporarily continue their insurance coverage, at the group rate received through their employer. Applies only to certain qualifying events: loss of job, reduction in hours worked, anticipation of legal separation or divorce, or loss of a spouse who has provided insurance.

Cognitive: Pertaining to thinking, understanding, learning, and logical thought.

Compartment syndrome: Compression of blood vessels from bleeding in one or more fascial compartments (enclosed spaces surrounding groups of organs or muscles, held together by sheets of connective tissue called fascia). Can lead to reduced blood flow to organs or muscles in the compartment, permanent nerve damage, and muscle death. SEE FASCIA.

Comprehensive care: Medical care that covers all aspects (mental, emotional, physical) of a patient's well-being and health. Comprehensive care team members for hemophilia include those from hematology, psychology, social services, dentistry, orthopedics, physical therapy.

Computed tomography (CT scan) or **computerized axial tomography** (CAT scan): Medical test that produces a cross-sectional x-ray image of the body. In hemophilia, sometimes used to detect internal bleeds, especially cranial bleeds.

Concentrate: SEE FACTOR CONCENTRATE.

CVAD: Central venous access device. SEE VENOUS ACCESS DEVICE.

Deep vein thrombosis (DVT): Blood clot that occurs in one of the large veins. DVT is a serious medical complication that happens relatively often in people using a CVAD.

Desmopressin acetate (DDAVP): Synthetic (manufactured) form of a hormone used to treat bleeding in people with mild hemophilia A. Not a clotting factor. Stimulates the release of factor VIII reserves into the blood to temporarily increase factor VIII levels.

Direct DNA mutational analysis (direct DNA test): A genetic carrier test. The hemophilia gene of an affected male is examined to determine the exact location and nature of the mutation that caused hemophilia in that person. If a specific mutation is identified, relatives can be screened to identify carrier status because the exact location of the mutation is known. A woman with the mutation is a carrier. SEE CARRIER TEST.

Glossary

DNA (deoxyribonucleic acid): Molecule that codes for how living organisms are built. Segments of DNA that give traits to offspring are called genes. SEE GENE.

EMLA: Brand name of a topical numbing cream. Effective in eliminating the pain of needlesticks. Must be applied to the needlestick site for 30–45 minutes before an infusion.

Enzymes: Proteins that are catalysts (capable of initiating or accelerating chemical reactions without being consumed).

EOB: Explanation of benefits. Documentation sent to patients by their insurance company that lists medical services received and reimbursed.

Event-related prophylaxis: Medical treatment for hemophilia that involves an infusion of factor concentrate given before an activity such as a sporting event or extended travel.

Factor: 1. One of the 13 blood proteins that help clot blood. 2. Informal term for any commercially prepared factor concentrate infused to replace the body's missing or inactive factor. SEE FACTOR CONCENTRATE.

Factor concentrate: Commercially prepared freeze-dried factor that is reconstituted with water or saline and infused to treat bleeding that results from factor deficiency.

Fascia: Strong sheets of connective tissue.

Fibrin: Protein required for blood clotting. Forms a net of fibers that hold blood platelets together in a clot, the end result of the clotting cascade.

Fibrin clot: Final result of the clotting cascade; a tough mesh of fibrin threads that weave through the platelet plug and form a blood clot to stop bleeding.

First generation: Classification of recombinant products. Introduced in 1992, these products use human or animal proteins in the growth medium. They also contain human albumin, added at the final production stage to help stabilize and bulk up the product.

Fractionation: Manufacturing process involving the separation of blood plasma into its various components such as clotting factors and human serum albumin.

Frenulum: Piece of skin that helps secure a mobile organ. Examples: the skin that bridges the inside of the upper lip to the gum; the skin that attaches the tongue to the floor of the mouth.

Gastrointestinal: Pertaining to the stomach or intestines.

Gene: Single unit of heredity. A segment of DNA that carries information for functional products such as proteins and is responsible for physical and inheritable traits of an organism such as hair color and eye color. Mutations (changes) to genes may cause genetic disorders such as hemophilia. Genes are sequences of DNA located in string-like groups called chromosomes, found in each cell. SEE CHROMOSOME.

Gene therapy: Procedure in which normally functioning genes can be inserted into a patient's own cells; in turn, those cells produce the specific protein controlled by the particular genes. Gene therapy is one area of research for a cure for hemophilia.

Genetic: Inherited.

Genetic mutation: Permanent change in a gene that scrambles the instructions carried by the gene. Hemophilia is a genetic mutation that scrambles the instructions for producing a blood-clotting protein such as factor VIII or IX.

Half-life: Time it takes for one-half of the clotting activity of infused factor to disappear. Factor VIII has a half-life of 8–12 hours; only half

Glossary

the factor is available 12 hours after being infused. Factor IX has a half-life of about 24 hours.

Heat treatment: Viral inactivation method that heats commercially prepared factor to destroy viruses. SEE PASTEURIZATION.

Hemarthrosis: Bleeding in a joint.

Hematoma: Tissue bleed; bruise.

Hematologist: Physician who studies the nature, function, and diseases of the blood.

Hematuria: Presence of blood in the urine.

Hemophilia: Any of several blood-clotting disorders in which excessive bleeding occurs because of the absence or abnormality of one of 13 clotting proteins called clotting factors. SEE FACTOR.

Hemophilia A (factor VIII deficiency, classic hemophilia): Blood-clotting disorder in which the factor VIII protein is missing or inactive.

Hemophilia B (Christmas disease): Blood-clotting disorder in which the factor IX protein is missing or inactive.

Hemophilia treatment center (HTC): Clinic staffed with a team of specialists who provide diagnosis, treatment, support, and information to people with bleeding disorders and their families.

Hemophilic arthropathy: Form of chronic arthritis in a person with hemophilia; caused by repeated bleeding into a joint.

Hemorrhage: Heavy or uncontrolled bleeding.

Hemostasis: Any process that causes bleeding to stop, whether biologically, as in the formation of a blood clot, or medically, as in surgery.

Hepatitis: Disease that causes inflammation and potential deterioration of the liver.

Hepatitis A (HAV): Disease that causes inflammation of the liver. Transmitted when people drink water, eat food, or touch objects contaminated by fecal matter from an HAV-infected person. Unlike hepatitis B and C, HAV doesn't usually cause chronic liver disease and is only rarely fatal. A vaccine is available. SEE APPENDIX D.

Hepatitis B (HBV): Disease that causes inflammation and potential deterioration of the liver. Transmitted through contact with infected blood or saliva; sexual contact with an infected person; IV drug use with contaminated needles; and, before viral inactivation methods, factor concentrates. Vaccines are available. SEE APPENDIX D.

Hepatitis C (HCV): Disease that causes inflammation and deterioration of the liver. Transmitted by direct contact with contaminated blood or blood products. Since 1985, when viral inactivation processes became available for factor concentrates, there have been no documented cases of HCV transmission through factor concentrates. There is no vaccine for HCV. SEE APPENDIX D.

Hereditary: Passing, or capable of passing, from parent to offspring naturally through the genes.

Home care company: Specialized contractor that provides certain medical services to patients in their homes, and can include a specialty pharmacy to distribute factor concentrate.

HTC: SEE HEMOPHILIA TREATMENT CENTER.

Human immunodeficiency virus (HIV): Virus that attacks the immune system and causes AIDS. Transmitted through contact with bodily fluids of an infected person, such as semen, blood, or mother's milk; and through sharing needles with an infected person. It takes three to six months after exposure before antibodies to the HIV virus appear in the bloodstream.

Iliopsoas (psoas): Large group of muscles in the hip area that help flex the thigh. Bleeding into this muscle group can result in compartment syndrome, causing numbness, loss of circulation, and death of muscles and nerves, possibly resulting in paralysis. SEE COMPARTMENT SYNDROME.

Immune system: Body's defense system that destroys foreign substances or viruses in the bloodstream.

Immune tolerance therapy (ITT): Therapy for inhibitor patients that requires high, frequent doses of factor concentrate to desensitize the body to factor VIII or IX infusions in the hope that, over time, the body may "learn" to recognize factor. SEE INHIBITOR.

Immunoadsorption: Purification technology typically used to remove antibodies from plasma. Example: the removal of inhibitors from plasma during plasmapheresis.

Immunoaffinity: Attraction of an antibody to an antigen. Some commercial plasma-derived factor concentrates are purified using monoclonal purification, a type of purification method using immunoaffinity in which **monoclonal antibodies** attract and remove factor VIII or IX (the antigen) from blood plasma. SEE MONOCLONAL ANTIBODY PURIFICATION.

Incidence: Frequency with which a disease or disorder appears in a certain population. Example: the incidence of hemophilia A is approximately 1 in 5,000 male births.

Indirect DNA linkage analysis (or restriction length fragment polymorphisms [RLFP]): Type of genetic carrier test in which DNA samples are compared from the potential carrier and from family members, some of whom are known to carry the hemophilia gene. Test detects differences that occur only in DNA associated with hemophilia. SEE DIRECT DNA MUTATIONAL ANALYSIS.

Infusion: Process of injecting reconstituted factor concentrate or another drug into the bloodstream through a vein.

Inhibitor: Antibody to factor VIII or IX. Inhibitors develop when the immune system identifies infused factor as a foreign material and produces antibodies to inactivate the factor.

Intermediate purity: One of several classifications of plasma-derived clotting factor; refers to the amount of extraneous (unwanted) proteins in the product.

Intracranial hemorrhage (ICH): Bleed inside the skull, usually caused by a head injury. Treated as a medical emergency.

Intravenous (IV): Infusion of liquid substances, such as factor concentrate, directly into a vein.

Jugular vein: One of several large veins in the neck that drain blood from the head.

Lipid: Fat; an important component of living cells. Also found in the outer layer of lipid-enveloped viruses, which are more susceptible than non-enveloped viruses to solvent-detergent wash used to inactivate viruses.

Lipid-enveloped virus: A virus with a lipid coat. SEE LIPID, NON-ENVELOPED VIRUS.

MASAC: Medical and Scientific Advisory Council of NHF. Makes recommendations about treatment and products to the US hemophilia community.

MedicAlert: 1. Nonprofit company that maintains a database of members' medical information that is made available to medical personnel during an emergency. 2. Brand name of medical identity bracelets or necklaces inscribed with pertinent information about a patient's disorder and treatment.

Medicaid: US government health insurance program financed by federal, state, and local funds to provide hospitalization and medical insurance for people of all ages who meet certain income limits.

Medicare: US government program of hospitalization insurance and voluntary medical insurance for people 65 and older, and for certain disabled people under 65.

Mild hemophilia: Classification of hemophilia in which the level of active factor is between 6% and 50%.

Moderate hemophilia: Classification of hemophilia in which the level of active factor is 1% to 5%.

Monoclonal antibodies: Group of identical antibodies that bind to a specific antigen, such as factor VIII or IX. Used in factor production to separate factor from blood plasma or, with recombinant products, from cell culture medium.

Monoclonal antibody purification: Immunoaffinity chromatography process used to produce some factor concentrates. As plasma or cell culture medium is poured through a column containing the antibodies, the antibodies attach to factor VIII or IX, pulling them out of the solution to concentrate and purify the clotting factors.

Multidisciplinary team: Medical team composed of several usually separate branches of learning or fields of expertise.

Mutation: Change in a gene or a chromosome that may cause death or disease, in rare cases.

Non-enveloped virus: Viruses that do not have a lipid (fatty) outer coating. Non-enveloped viruses are highly resistant to viral inactivation processes. SEE LIPID, ENVELOPED VIRUS.

Obligate carrier: Person who carries the gene of a specific trait by default. In hemophilia, a female is an obligate carrier if her father had hemophilia, she has more than one son with hemophilia, or she has one son and another blood relative with hemophilia.

Parvovirus (HPV) B19: Non-enveloped virus that is highly resistant to current viral inactivation methods used on factor concentrates. Parvovirus infection usually doesn't lead to serious illness but can cause short-term arthropathy.

Pasteurization: Viral inactivation method that involves heating commercially prepared factor in a liquid state to destroy viruses.

Payer: Entity that reimburses the cost of medical services and products. Can include private insurance companies, public programs such as Medicaid and Medicare, and certain state programs.

PBM: SEE PHARMACY BENEFIT MANAGER.

Percutaneous blood sampling (PUBS): Type of carrier test that provides information about the risk of certain blood disorders, such as hemophilia. Performed after week 20 of pregnancy, PUBS involves removing a sample of fetal blood from the umbilical vein, with results available in a few days.

Peripheral: Near the surface or outside of; external. Peripheral veins in the hands or elbow are often used for factor infusions.

Pharmacokinetic study (PK study): Study of the effects and behavior of a drug in the body.

Pharmacy benefit manager (PBM): Company hired by insurance companies to manage insurance benefits and prescription drug plans of private-sector entities such as employers, labor unions, and managed care companies. PBMs help determine the formulary (a listing of drugs that a payer will reimburse) and help keep prescription drug costs low for the insurance company.

PHS pricing (340B Drug Pricing Program): Government program that allows federally funded HTCs to purchase factor from pharmaceutical companies at a significant discount.

Plasma: Liquid part of blood. Contains factors VIII and IX, and von Willebrand factor.

Plasma derived: Term used to describe factor concentrate made from human blood plasma.

Plasmapheresis: Process of harvesting a patient's plasma by continuously removing the blood, separating the blood cells, and returning the cells to the patient. Plasma is collected and frozen for use in producing medications such as factor concentrate. Plasmapheresis may also be used to temporarily reduce inhibitors by passing the plasma through an immunoadsorption column and then returning it to the patient.

Platelets: Plate-shaped cell fragments in the bloodstream that create a plug over an injury site in a blood vessel wall. Platelets are essential for blood clotting.

Platelet plug: The sticky accumulation of platelets that occurs when platelets are activated at the site of a blood vessel injury as the body attempts to stem bleeding. One step in the coagulation process.

Porcine: Related to pigs. In the past, porcine factor VIII concentrate was used to treat bleeds in hemophilia A patients with inhibitors.

Port: Central venous access device surgically implanted under the skin, typically in the chest wall, to facilitate IV infusions. SEE CENTRAL VENOUS ACCESS DEVICE.

Possible carrier: Person who may carry a gene for a specific trait, such as hemophilia. Possible carriers in hemophilia include mothers of children with hemophilia who have no history of hemophilia in the family and daughters of carrier mothers.

Prenatal testing: Medical testing done during pregnancy, often to check for genetic disorders or birth defects.

Prevalence: Number of cases of a disorder or disease present in a given population at a certain time. The prevalence of people with hemophilia in the United States is estimated to be about 20,000.

Primary prophylaxis: Medical treatment for hemophilia that involves scheduled infusions of factor concentrate before any joint damage occurs, and sometimes even before any bleeds occur, usually in infancy.

Prolonged half-life: Describes commercial recombinant factor concentrate modified to maintain clotting activity for an extended period past the normal half-life of the particular factor.

Prophylaxis: Medical treatment for hemophilia that involves scheduled infusions of factor concentrate. Designed to keep factor levels high enough in the bloodstream to prevent most, if not all, spontaneous bleeds.

Prothrombin complex concentrate (PCC): Bypassing agent used to control bleeding in patients with inhibitors. SEE ACTIVATED PROTHROMBIN COMPLEX CONCENTRATE, INHIBITOR, BYPASSING AGENT.

Protocol: Plan for carrying out a scientific study or a patient's treatment regimen.

Purification: Production processes designed to reduce the quantity of foreign proteins in factor concentrates that may cause allergic reactions. Monoclonal antibody purification is one such process.

Purity: Amount of foreign proteins present in factor concentrates; usually expressed as a ratio of the amount of clotting factor present per milligram of protein. A higher purity number means more clotting factor and less unwanted protein.

Recall: Removal of a medical product from the market when it violates FDA requirements. May be initiated when products are not stored at correct temperatures, are not manufactured according to their approved specifications, are labeled incorrectly, or are not as potent as labeled. SEE WITHDRAWAL.

Recombinant factor: Factor concentrate produced from genetically engineered mammal cells containing the human gene for factor. The human factor gene is spliced into a mammalian cell, instructing the cell to produce human factor. Recombinant factor does not carry blood-borne viruses.

Recombinant factor VIIa: Activated recombinant factor VII. ("Activated" means that the factor doesn't need to be triggered by another clotting factor to do its job.) This effective alternative treatment for bleeds in people with inhibitors is a type of bypassing therapy because activated factor VII helps to create a clot—by activating factor X—without the need for factor VIII or IX.

Reconstitution: Process of returning freeze-dried, powdered factor concentrates to a liquid state by mixing with sterile water or sterile saline solution.

Reconstitution device: Any of various medical ancillaries used to reconstitute factor without using needles.

Recovery study: Test to determine the amount of factor circulating in the bloodstream after an infusion of factor. SEE PHARMACOKINETIC STUDY.

Regimen: A regulated course, as of diet, exercise, manner of living, or medical treatment, intended to preserve or restore health or attain some result.

Safety: Manufacturing measures taken to remove potentially harmful substances, including viruses, from factor concentrate.

Second generation: Classification of recombinant products. No human albumin is added to the final product, but human or animal proteins are used in the growth medium.

Secondary prophylaxis: Medical treatment for hemophilia that involves scheduled infusions of factor concentrate after a child has already experienced one or more bleeds into a single joint and before a target joint develops.

Serum: Blood plasma without clotting factors.

Severe hemophilia: Classification of hemophilia in which the level of active factor is less than 1%.

Severity level: Hemophilia classification system based on the percentage of normal factor active in the blood. There are three severity levels: severe, moderate, and mild. Severe hemophilia: less than 1% of factor is active. Moderate hemophilia: 1% to 5% of factor is active. Mild hemophilia: more than 6% to 50% of factor is active. Normal factor activity is considered to be between 50% and 150%, with most people near 100%.

Sharps: Generic name for commercial hard containers used for the safe disposal of needles and other sharp medical instruments.

Solvent-detergent wash (SD): Viral inactivation method that destroys lipid-enveloped viruses such as hepatitis B, hepatitis C, HIV, while leaving the factor VIII protein intact and functional.

Sonogram: Picture produced by an ultrasound exam. SEE ULTRASOUND.

Specialty pharmacy: Licensed distributor of biologic products such as factor concentrates.

Spontaneous bleeds: Bleeds that occur with no apparent injury. Usually experienced by people with severe hemophilia.

Sterile: Free of microorganisms. Examples: surgical instruments, infusion needles, and syringes are sterile before the package is opened.

Subcutaneous: Under the skin. All inoculations should be given subcutaneously in children with hemophilia.

Glossary

Symptomatic carrier: Carrier who exhibits excessive bleeding. Symptomatic carriers essentially have hemophilia and risk excessive bleeding during dental extraction, surgery, or childbirth, and may have frequent nosebleeds, bruising, and heavy menstrual bleeding.

Syndrome: Group of symptoms and diseases that together indicate a specific disease or medical condition.

Synovitis: Inflammation of the synovium in a joint. May contribute to more frequent joint bleeds and development of a target joint.

Synovium: Thin layer of connective tissue that lines the cavity of a joint. Produces synovial fluid, which lubricates the joints. Joint bleeds irritate the synovium, causing synovitis.

Syringe: Small tube with a plunger used for IV infusions and injections.

Target joint: Joint that repeatedly bleeds. Over time, target joints will develop arthritis.

Tertiary prophylaxis: Medical treatment for hemophilia that involves scheduled infusions of factor concentrate after a person has developed a target joint. SEE TARGET JOINT.

Third generation: Classification of recombinant products, first available in 2003, containing no human or animal proteins in the growth medium or added to the final product. These products have the lowest risk of transmitting viruses.

Thrombosis: Unwanted blood clot in the circulatory system, as in the heart, arteries, veins, capillaries.

Titer: Laboratory measurement of the amount of a substance in a solution. In hemophilia, titer most often refers to inhibitor antibody level. SEE BETHESDA UNIT.

Tourniquet: Strip of rubber or other material secured around the arm or leg to restrict blood flow, allowing veins to become more prominent before venipuncture.

Triage: Process of sorting patients who need immediate treatment based on medical priority.

Trough level: Lowest level of active factor in the bloodstream between prophylactic infusions.

Ultrapure: One of several purity classifications of commercial plasma-derived factor. Factor concentrates purified using monoclonal antibodies are ultrapure.

Ultrasound: Medical imaging method using high-frequency sound waves to produce images of structures within the body. SEE SOUNOGRAM.

Vasoconstriction: Automatic narrowing of a blood vessel to reduce the flow of blood, for example, in response to an injury.

Veins: Blood vessels that bring blood back to the heart from all parts of the body. IV medications are typically infused into veins.

Venipuncture: Insertion of a needle into a vein.

Viral inactivation: Manufacturing safety process used during factor production that makes blood-borne viruses, such as HIV and hepatitis, non-infective through the use of heat or solvent-detergent wash.

von Willebrand disease (VWD): Most common inherited bleeding disorder. Caused by low levels of von Willebrand factor (VWF) or malfunctioning VWF; results in platelets not sticking together during blood clotting. Symptoms include prolonged bleeding, nosebleeds, soft tissue bleeds, menorrhagia, gastrointestinal bleeds. VWD affects men and women equally, but is diagnosed more often in women because of bleeding problems in childbirth and menstruation.

Glossary

von Willebrand factor (VWF): Blood protein that circulates bound to factor VIII. VWF is believed to help stabilize factor VIII and carry it to bleeding sites. Patients with VWD are deficient in VWF and show decreased factor VIII activity.

Withdrawal: Voluntary removal from the market, or correction, of an FDA-regulated product found to be out of compliance with FDA regulations when the FDA would not pursue legal action. Products can be withdrawn during normal stock rotation; routine equipment adjustment and repair; product improvement; or as a result of actual or alleged tampering with individual units, providing there is no evidence of manufacturing or distribution problems. SEE RECALL.

X chromosome: X-shaped chromosome that carries the gene with instructions for female development. One of the two sex chromosome, along with the Y chromosome found in males. Any gene on the X chromosome, including the hemophilia gene, is said to be X-linked.

Y chromosome: Y-shaped chromosome that carries the gene with instructions for male development. Found only in males. Along with the X, the Y is one of the two sex chromosomes.

Index

Some terms appear throughout the text (for example, factor). For those terms, only major subtopics are indexed. In some cases, entire chapters are devoted to specific topics (for example, Chapter 7, Prophylax—and Relax!). For those chapters, only selected page references may be included in the index.

A

acetaminophen, 81, 90, 334; defined 339
acetylsalicylic acid (ASA), 81, 334; defined 341
acquired hemophilia, 293 ch. 2 n.2, 299 ch. 14 n.1; defined 339
acquired immune deficiency syndrome (AIDS), 19; defined 339
activated prothrombin complex concentrate (aPCC), 238, 243; defined 339
aerobic activity, 190
Affordable Care Act (ACA), 245, 265; defined 339
AIDS: see acquired immune deficiency syndrome
albumin, 96, 97, 99, 100 fig. 6.2, 296 ch. 6 n.6 & 7, 333; defined 340
allergic reaction, 159, 238; see also anaphylaxis
Amicar, 45, 78, 79, 90, 154-55, 294 ch. 3 n.5, 295 ch. 5 n.3, 338; defined 340
amniocentesis, 221, 222, 223, 228, 298 ch. 12 n.7; defined 340
analgesic, 295 ch. 5 n.7; defined 340
anamnestic response, 235, 238, 299 ch. 14 n.12; defined 340
anaphylaxis, 159, 294 ch. 3 n.7, 332; defined 340; see also allergic reaction
ancillaries, 106, 108, 109, 162, 163, 166; defined 340
anemia, 45, 51; defined 340
anesthesia
    circumcision and, 38-39
    ports and, 122
antibody 243
    defined, 341

tests for, 326-27
antifibrinolytic, 45; defined 341
antigen, 326, 333 App. D. n.4; defined 341
aPCC: *see* activated prothrombin complex concentrate
arthritis, 47-48, 153
arthropathy, 48 fig. 3.1; defined 341; *see also* hemophilic arthropathy
aseptic, 123, 125, 127, 158; defined 341
aspirin: *see* acetylsalicylic acid
assay, 102-103, 104, 106, 108; *see also* Bethesda inhibitor assay
aura, 127, 153

B

baseline factor level test, 220, 224
Bethesda inhibitor assay, 235, 299 ch. 14 n.8
Bethesda titer: *see* Bethesda unit
Bethesda unit (BU), 235, 243; defined 341
bleeding pattern, 44, 118, 119, 120, 151, 152, 153, 156, 166, 257
blood-borne virus, 96, 98, 111, 324
    hepatitis A and, 329
blood clot, 20-23
    mouth and, 78
    ports and, 125
    risks of, 123
    thrombosis and, 124, 214, 239
blood vessel
    bruising and, 76-77
    explained, 20-23
brand restriction, 253
breakthrough bleed, 117-18, 153, 241; defined 342
Broviac, 121, 338
bruise, 76-77
    environment and, 85
    head bleed and, 52, 226, 228

infusions and, 85
  needlestick and, 40
  others' reactions to, 170, 172, 175, 208
  throat bleed and, 50
  treatment for, 44-45
BU: see Bethesda unit
bullies, 177-78, 181
bypassing agent, 236-37; defined 342

C

capillaries, 20; defined 342
capitation, 250
carrier (hemophilia), 18, 25, 139
  birth and, 221-25, 227, 228
  defined, 342
  feelings about being, 5, 6, 7, 204
  inheritance of, 31-35, 213-17, 293 ch. 1 n.3, 293 ch. 2 n.7, 298
    ch. 13 n.2 & 5
  status of, 62, 214-19, 221, 228
  test for, 34, 62, 217-20, 294 ch. 2 n.8; defined 342
  See also possible carrier
car seat, 84, 164
cartilage, 47, 55, 114, 153
cauterization, 41; defined 342
CDC: see Centers for Disease Control and Prevention
Centers for Disease Control and Prevention (CDC), 164, 185, 293 ch. 2 n.1
central venous access device (CVAD), 113, 121-22, 124; defined 342;
  see also port
chest pain, 158
childbirth, 215, 219, 220, 226, 292 ch. 1 n.2
Children's Health Insurance Program (CHIP), 266-67
CHIP: see Children's Health Insurance Program
chorionic villus sampling (CVS), 221, 222-23; defined 342

363

Christmas disease, 24; defined 343; *see also* hemophilia B
chromatography, 96; defined 343
chromosome
    defined, 343
    hemophilia inheritance and, 30-34, 219
    inactivation and, 32, 33
    sex and, 7, 30-32, 214
circumcision, 37, 38-40, 41, 225, 294 ch. 3 n.2; defined 343
CJD: *see* Creutzfeldt-Jakob disease
clotting cascade, 21-23; defined 343
clotting factor, 22
    defined, 343
    factor concentrate and, 237-38, 299 ch. 14 n.10, 324
    functional clotting factor, 32
    hemophilia and, 19, 24, 31-32, 34, 35, 214, 230
    infusion and, 26, 28, 129
    prophylaxis and, 129
    purity and, 96
COBRA: *see* Consolidated Omnibus Budget Reconciliation Act
coinsurance, 254, 255, 256, 258
compartment syndrome, 42, 46, 49; defined 344
compassionate care programs, 270, 271
comprehensive care, 58, 74; defined 344
computed tomography (CT), 59, 294 ch. 3 n.8; defined 344
Consolidated Omnibus Budget Reconciliation Act (COBRA), 265, 266-67, 268, 271; defined 343
copayment, 248
corporal punishment, 141-42, 143; *see also* discipline
Creutzfeldt-Jakob disease (CJD), 328, 329, 330-32
C-section, 220, 224
CSHCNP: *see* Children with Special Healthcare Needs Programs
CT scan: *see* computed tomography
CVS: *see* chronic villus sampling

D

DDAVP: *see* desmopressin acetate
deductible, 249, 251, 253, 254, 255, 256, 259
deep vein thrombosis (DVT), 124, 125; defined 344
dental work, 49
desmopressin acetate (DDAVP), 27, 35, 219-20, 338; defined 344
diagnostic tests, 62, 250, 252
    HIV and, 325-27
diluent, 28
direct DNA mutational analysis (direct DNA test), 217, 218; defined 344; *see also* carrier, indirect DNA linkage analysis
discipline, 141-45, 150, 178, 194
distributor
    factor, 93 fig. 6.1
    HTC as, 106-107
dizziness, 52, 158
DNA, 222, 299 ch. 14 n.4
    defined, 345
    sequencing of, 30
    testing, 217-19
dosage
    factor and, 70, 118, 119
    factor VIII and, 336
    factor IX and, 337
    understanding of, 63, 158, 166
Drug Pricing Program, 107; *see also* Public Health Service
DTaP vaccine, 53
DVT: *see* deep vein thrombosis

E

emergency room, use of, 42, 57, 69-71
EMLA, 88, 295 ch. 5 n.9, 338; defined 345
EOB: *see* explanation of benefits

epinephrine, 159
EpiPen, 159, 338
EPO: *see* exclusive provider organization
ER: *see* emergency room
event-related prophylaxis, 117, 129; defined 315
exclusive provider organization (EPO), 251
explanation of benefits (EOB), 258-59, 263; defined 345
external devices, 121-22
eye bleed, 51

F
factor VII, 101
factor VIII
    bypassing agents for, 237-38
    deficiency of, 24, 27, 118, 219, 232, 243
    dosage calculation for, 336-37
    half-life of, 29-30, 119
    inhibitor and, 229-31, 232-33, 237-238, 240-41, 243, 299 ch. 14 n.1 & 4
    prophylactic infusion for, 118
    See also acquired hemophilia, carrier, factor concentrate, hemophilia A, porcine factor VIII
factor IX
    bypassing agents for, 237-38
    deficiency of, 24, 27
    dosage calculation for, 336-37
    half-life of, 29-30, 118
    inhibitor and, 229, 232, 237, 240-41, 243
    nanofiltration and, 99
    prophylactic infusion for, 118
    See also carrier, Christmas disease, factor concentrate, hemophilia B

factor activity level, 29 fig. 2.2, 152
factor brands, 103 table 6.1
factor concentrate, 237–39, 299 ch. 14 n.10
    freeze-dried, 28
    purity and, 94–101, 104, 112, 295 ch. 6 n.3, 324–30; defined 354
factor delivery, 91, 109
factor protein, 94, 96, 242
factor replacement therapy, 27, 28, 35, 219–20
family planning, 34, 296 ch. 6 n.10
    carrier status and, 214, 216, 227
Fee-for-Service (FFS), 248–49
fever, 81, 90, 123, 158, 295 ch. 5 n.7, 329
FFS: *see* Fee-for-Service
fibrin, 22, 23 fig. 2.1, 124; defined 345
    clot, 21, 22, 24, 27, 35; defined 345
forceps, 223, 224, 225
foreskin, 38; *see also* circumcision
formulary, 109, 253, 256, 300 ch. 15 n.5
fractionation, 327, 328, 332; defined 346
frenulum, 77, 90; defined 346

G

gastrointestinal (GI) tract
    bleed, 49, 51, 153, 155–56
    defined, 345
gene therapy, defined 346
genetic disorder, 17, 30, 35
genetically engineered cells, 94, 98
geneticist, 34, 59, 216, 218
GI bleed: *see* gastrointestinal tract – bleed
gum bleed, 79, 153, 154, 156

H

half-life of factor, 29, 119, 235, 299 ch. 14 n.6
- defined, 346
- factor VIII, 29, 118
- factor IX, 29–30, 118
- low-responding inhibitor and, 236
- prolonged, 30, 95, 101, 102, 110, 112, 118

HANDI, 14, 242, 293 ch. 1 n.4, 298 ch. 11 n.7

head bleed, 49, 51–52, 63
- infants and, 223, 225–26, 228, 294 ch. 3 n.8

head bump, 63, 79, 82, 85, 90, 294 ch. 4 n.3, 295 ch. 5 n.5

health maintenance organization (HMO), 250, 251, 296 ch. 6 n.9

health savings account (HSA), 257–58

helmet, 19, 51, 83, 188, 189, 207, 298 ch. 11 n.6

hemarthrosis, 45; defined 347; *see also* joint bleed

hematologist, defined 347

hematoma, 40, defined 347; *see also* bruise

hematuria, 155; defined 347

hemophilia A, 17, 24, 27, 31, 35, 293 ch. 2 n.1, 298 ch. 13 n.3
- carriers and, 220
- defined, 347
- inhibitors and, 233, 236, 238

hemophilia B (Christmas disease), 17, 24, 25, 31, 118, 293 ch. 2 n.1
- allergic reactions and, 159
- defined, 347
- inhibitors and, 236, 238
- pregnancy and, 220

Hemophilia Federation of America (HFA), 14, 262, 297 ch. 10 n.1, 333

hemophilia, inheritance of, 2, 30–34, 206

hemophilia, myths about, 18–20, 170

hemophilia, severity of; *see* mild hemophilia, moderate hemophilia, severe hemophilia

hemophilia treatment center (HTC), defined 347
hemophilic arthropathy, 47-48, 153; defined 347; *see also* arthopathy
hemorrhage, defined 347; *see also* intracranial hemorrhage
hemostasis, 21-22; defined 347
hepatitis, 98, 325; defined 347
    hepatitis A (HAV), 53, 98, 296 ch. 6 n.5, 327, 329; defined 347-48
    hepatitis B (HBV), 53, 98, 296 ch. 6 n.7, 298 ch. 13 n.10, 327, 328, 329; defined 348
    hepatitis C (HCV), 98, 104, 111, 296 ch. 6 n.7, 324, 327, 328; defined 348
HFA: *see* Hemophilia Federation of America
hib vaccine, 53
Hickman, 121, 338
high-titer inhibitor, 235, 236, 238, 243, 299 ch. 14 n.8 & 9
HIV: *see* human immunodeficiency virus
hives, 158
HMO: *see* health maintenance organization
home care company, 105, 107
    defined, 348
    self-infusion and, 281
    services and, 105, 108, 112, 160, 253, 254, 257, 261, 262, 270, 281
    travel and, 162, 164, 297 ch. 9 n.8
home infusion, 157, 158-59, 160, 161, 165, 210, 254, 257, 296 ch. 7 n.2
hospital pharmacy, 104, 105
human immunodeficiency virus (HIV), 19-20, 98, 296 ch. 6 n.7
    blood supply and, 20, 111, 324-27
    defined, 348
    factor concentrate and, 104

I

ICH: *see* intracranial hemorrhage
iliopsoas, 49; defined 348

immune system
    antibody and, 229, 326
    bacteria and, 123
    defined, 349
    inhibitor and, 229, 231, 234, 235, 238, 240, 243, 296 ch. 7 n.3, 299 ch. 14 n.1, 10 & 12
immune tolerance therapy (ITT), 240; defined 349
immunization: see vaccination, vaccine
immunoadsorption, 239; defined 349
immunoaffinity, 98; defined 349
incidence
    defined, 349
    inhibitors and, 231-34
indirect DNA linkage analysis, 217, 218-19; defined 349; see also carrier, direct DNA mutational analysis
individual bleeding pattern, 118, 151, 153
infants
    birth and, 223, 225-26, 298 ch. 13 n.8
    bleeds and, 46, 52, 78-79, 80-81, 298 ch. 13 n.9
    bruising and, 76-77
    circumcision and, 39, 55
    fever and, 81
    immune tolerance therapy and, 240-41
    immunization schedule and, 53
    MedicAlert and, 84
    needlestick and, 86
    teething and, 77
    vaccination and, 40
    weight and, 186
    See also childbirth
infection
    blood product safety and, 324, 325, 326, 327, 329, 330
    circumcision and, 38, 39
    human immunodeficiency virus (HIV) and, 19-20

    infusion and, 158, 282, 296 ch. 7 n.3
    needlestick and, 164
    percutaneous blood sampling (PUBS) and, 223
    port and, 123-127, 128, 129, 241
    urinary tract bleed and, 154-55
infusion, xiii, 26
    allergy and, 159
    birth and, 224, 226
    bleed and, 44, 45, 49, 78-79, 154, 155
    camp and, 192-93, 195, 196
    charts of, 160-61, 166, 259
    children's behavior and, 123, 134, 140, 145-48, 198-200, 208
    circumcision and, 39, 294 ch. 3 n.2
    defined, 349
    factor and, 27, 28-30, 35, 233, 234, 235, 236
    infants and, 85-90
    medical treatment and, 62-63, 64, 67, 68, 69, 70-71, 73, 295 ch. 4 n.7, 295 ch. 5 n.9
    needlestick and, 65
    port and, 122, 123, 126, 127, 128, 129
    prophylaxis and, 26, 113, 114, 116-21
    school and, 173, 297 ch. 10 n.2
    teenagers and, 274, 276, 281, 283, 285, 288
    travel and, 162
    See also Bethesda unit, factor, home infusion, inhibitor, self-infusion
inherited trait, 30
inhibitor, defined 350; *see also* factor
in-network, 106, 108, 250, 251
intermediate purity, 95, 100, 112, 295 ch. 6 n.3; defined 350
internal device: *see* central venous access device
intracranial hemorrhage (ICH), 59, 126, 226, 298 ch. 13 n.9; defined 350
intravenous, 28; defined 350
ITT: *see* immune tolerance therapy

J

joint, 47
    growth of, 154
    injury prevention for, 83, 183, 184, 185–86, 189–90, 196
    medical care for, 59, 62, 71, 72
    See also arthropathy, factor, hemarthrosis, joint bleed, joint damage
joint bleed, 26, 47–48, 55, 81–82
    inhibitor and, 230, 241
    infusion and, 85
    prophylaxis and, 26, 113–15, 117, 120–21, 126, 129, 287
    symptoms of, 47, 48
    target joint and, 117, 119, 120–21, 126, 152, 153–54, 166; defined 357
    types of, 44–46, 50 fig. 3.2
joint damage 17, 47, 48 fig. 3.1
jugular vein, 68; defined 350

K

kidney bleed, 154–55, 295 ch. 5 n.3

L

labor and delivery, 224–25
lipid, viruses and, 328, 329, 333 App. D n.6; defined, 350
L.M.X.4, 88, 295 ch. 5 n.9, 338
low-titer inhibitor, 235, 236, 237, 239

M

mail-order pharmacy, 104, 109, 253
major bleed, 27, 45, 55
    inhibitor risk and, 234
    repeated, 114
managed care, 248, 249–51
MASAC: *see* Medical and Scientific Advisory Council

Medicaid, 246, 247, 263, 266, 267, 268, 295 ch. 6 n.1, 296 ch. 6 n.10, 297 ch. 9 n.7
    circumcision coverage and, 39
    defined, 350
    factor and, 247 fig. 15.1
Medical and Scientific Advisory Council (MASAC), 53, 100, 104, 111, 114, 225, 261, 333 App. D n.3; defined 350
medical benefit, insurance and, 252, 253
medical insurance
    employment and, 286
    travel and, 165, 166
    See also Medicaid, Medicare
Medicare, 246, 247, 253, 263, 267, 268, 295 ch. 6 n.1, 296 ch. 6 n.10
    defined, 351
    factor and, 247 fig. 15.1
mild hemophilia, 24-25, 34, 35, 47, 220
    carriers and, 215, 217, 219, 294 ch. 2 n.7
    defined, 351
    inhibitor and, 236
    nosebleed and, 154
    prophylaxis and, 115, 118
minor bleed, 27, 39, 44-45, 55
miscarriage, 221, 222, 223, 298 ch. 13 n.7
MMR vaccine, 53
moderate hemophilia, 25, 26-27, 35, 47
    birth and, 226
    bleeding pattern and, 152, 156
    defined, 351
    ICH and, 224
    infusion and, 147, 195, 231
    prophylaxis and, 119
monoclonal
    antibodies, defined 351

antibody purification, defined 351
factor concentrate and, 100 fig. 6.2
purity, 95, 96, 99, 112
viruses and, 98
mouth bleed, 44, 46, 50, 82, 155-56
treatment for, 45, 77-78
MRI, 63, 226, 297 ch. 7 n.4
multidisciplinary team, 12; defined 351
muscle bleed, 42, 45, 46, 49, 50 fig. 3.2, 55, 80
bleeding pattern and, 153, 156, 166
iliopsoas and, 49
infusion and, 85
mutation, 31, 293 ch. 1 n.3, 298 ch. 12 n.3
defined, 351
inhibitors and, 231, 233, 299 ch. 14 n.3
tests for, 216, 217-18
types of, 34, 233

N

nanofiltration, 99, 328
National Hemophilia Foundation (NHF), 14
neck bleed, 51
nerve damage, 49
NHF: see National Hemophilia Foundation
non-random X chromosome inactivation, 32
nosebleed, 44, 46, 50, 154
bleeding pattern and, 153, 166
carrier status and, 217, 219
treatment for, 45, 78, 155-56
nurse
camp, 192, 193, 195
coordinator, 58, 59, 60, 156, 161

ER triage, 70, 72
home care, 106, 157, 254
pediatric, 43
school, 169, 170, 173–74, 181, 297 ch. 10 n.2

O

obesity, 185, 282
obligate carrier, 215, 228; defined 351
on-demand therapy, 115, 120, 126, 127, 254, 296 ch. 7 n.2 & 3
open enrollment period, 253, 255, 256
orphan drug, 93, 295 ch. 6 n.2
orthopedist, 59, 60, 158, 184
out-of-network, 250, 251
overprotection, 137–38, 150, 171, 181, 206, 209, 242, 279

P

pain
    allergic reaction and, 158
    bruises and, 77
    circumcision and, 38, 39
    deep vein thrombosis and, 297 ch. 7 n.4
    eye bleed and, 51
    feelings about, vii, 2, 86, 137, 204, 241
    gastrointestinal bleed and, 51
    hepatitis A and, 329
    hepatitis B and, 329
    infusion and, 145, 153, 157
    inhibitors and, 242
    joint bleed and, 47, 48 fig. 3.1, 153
    medical treatment for, 64, 68, 69, 71, 72
    medications for, 81, 295 ch. 5 n.7 & 9

major bleed and, 45-46, 55
mouth bleed and, 46
muscle bleed and, 42, 49
prophylaxis and, 114
punishment and, 143
throat bleed and, 50
urinary tract bleed and, 155

parvovirus, 296 ch. 6 n.5, 327, 329; defined 352
pasteurization, 98, 328, 333 App. D n.6; defined 352
Patient Services Inc. (PSI), 269-70
payer, 92, 93 fig. 6.1, 102, 104, 111, 246, 247, 248, 253, 263, 295 ch. 6 n.1
    defined, 352
    HMO as, 250
    HTC and, 106
    pharmacy benefit manager and, 109
    recordkeeping and, 258-59
    specialty pharmacies and, 105, 106

PBM: *see* pharmacy benefit manager
PCP: *see* primary care physician
PDL: *see* preferred drug list
pediatrician
    blood work and, 80
    bruising care and, 76
    childbirth care and, 225
    coughing care and, 80
    ER care and, 70
    HTC and, 58
    needlestick care and, 40, 55, 88, 298 ch. 12 n.10

penis: *see* circumcision
percutaneous blood sampling (PUBS), 221, 223, 270; defined 352
pharmaceutical company/manufacturer: 92, 93 fig. 6.1, 101, 107, 109, 257, 261, 262, 270, 300 ch. 16 n.3, 317
pharmacy benefit, 248, 252, 253, 256
pharmacy benefit manager (PBM), 109, 248; defined 352

PHS: see Public Health Service
physical therapist, 59, 187, 193
plasma
    bypassing agents and, 237-38
    bypassing procedures and, 239
    clotting and, 21, 22
    defined, 353
    inhibitors and, 235, 299 ch. 14 n.7
    See also Bethesda unit, immunoadsorption, plasma-derived factor concentrate, plasmapheresis
plasma-derived factor concentrate, 94-95, 100, 101, 103 table 6.1, 112, 296 ch. 6 n.6, 324
    defined, 353
    purity and, 96, 99, 327, 333 App. D n.2, 3 & 6
    safety of, 111, 324-25, 327, 332-33
    viral inactivation and, 99, 327-29
    See also factor concentrate – purity, plasma
plasmapheresis, 239, 325, 330; defined 353
platelet, 21, 22
    aspirin and, 81
    deep vein thrombosis and, 124
    defined, 353
    NSAIDs and, 81
    porcine factor VIII and, 238
    von Willebrand disease and, 293 ch. 2 n.4
platelet plug, 21, 22, 23 fig. 2.1, 35, 81; defined 353
play therapy, 146, 147-48, 150
pneumococcal vaccine, 53
point-of-service (POS), 251
porcine factor VIII, 238; defined 353
port, defined 353; see also central venous access device, infusion
POS: see point-of-service
possible carrier, 215-16; defined 353

postnatal tests, 226
PPO: see preferred provider organization
preferred provider organization (PPO), 246, 251, 253
prenatal testing, 221-23, 228
prevalence, 231-32, 243; defined 354
price per unit, 103, 107, 110, 248
primary care physician (PCP), 165, 249
primary prophylaxis, 117, 129; defined 354; see also prophylaxis
prolonged half-life: see half-life of factor - prolonged
prophylaxis
    bleeds and, 55, 79, 83, 113, 114, 152, 153-54
    CVADs and, 121-22
    defined, 354
    immunizations and, 42
    physical activity and, 187
    purpose of, 26, 117-19
    risk factors of, 233
    treatment and insurance, 254, 263
    weaning from, 127, 285, 287
    See also event-related prophylaxis, primary prophylaxis,
      secondary prophylaxis, tertiary prophylaxis
protective gear, 19, 83, 188-89, 196, 277
prothrombin complex concentrate (PCC), 237-38; defined 354
PSI: see Patient Services Inc.
psoas: see iliopsoas
public assistance, 268, 269, 271
Public Health Service (PHS), 105, 107, 296 ch. 6 n.10
    PHS pricing defined, 353
PUBS: see percutaneous blood sampling
punishment: see discipline

Q

Queen Victoria, 18

R

R.I.C.E., 298 ch. 11 n.5
radiologist, 59
recall, product, 160; defined 354
recombinant factor concentrate, 94–97, 102–103, 104, 112, 242, 324
    defined, 355
    factor VII, 101
    factor VIIa, 238, 243; defined 355
    factor VIII, 101
    first generation, 99, 100, 112; defined 346
    manufacturers of, 101, 103 table 6.1
    pricing of, 104, 110
    purity of, 99, 100
    second generation, 97, 100, 112; defined 355
    third generation, 97, 98, 100, 112; defined 357
    viral inactivation and, 99, 111, 296 ch. 6 n.6, 296 ch. 7 n.1, 300 ch. 15 n.5, 324
reconstitution, 28, 103, 163; defined 355
reimbursement
    claim denial and, 261
    HTC and, 269
    insurance and, 248, 258
    specialty pharmacies and, 106, 109

S

safety
    blood products and, 20, 111, 296 ch. 6 n.6, 324, 332–33
    defined, 355
    infusions and, 119
    purity and, 95, 96, 97, 104, 112
    sports and, 190
    teaching about, 137, 138–39, 150, 188, 280, 281, 282
    See also protective gear

saline, 28
saliva, 78, 79, 329
SD: *see* solvent-detergent wash
seasonal bleed, 156
seatbelt, 84, 164, 283
secondary prophylaxis, 117, 119; defined 356; *see also* prophylaxis
self-infusion
    adolescents and, 283
    camp and, 193, 195, 196
severe bleed, 49, 55, 220, 296 ch. 7 n.3, 337
severe hemophilia, 25, 49
    bleeds and, 26, 27, 47, 152
    defined, 356
    HIV and, 19–20
    inhibitors and, 232, 233, 234, 236
    mutations and, 233, 298 ch. 13 n.3
    non-random X chromosome and, 32
    prophylaxis and, 118, 119, 120
    self-infusion and, 195
    treatment of, 78, 154, 294 ch. 3 n.5
severity level: *see* mild hemophilia, moderate hemophilia, severe hemophilia
shock
    emotional response, 1, 4–5, 12, 15, 39, 78, 205, 223, 230
    physical response, 45, 51
shortness of breath: *see* allergic reaction
Social Security Disability Income (SSDI), 269, 271
solvent-detergent (SD) wash, 98, 296 ch. 6 n.5, 328, 329, 330, 333 App. D n.6; defined 356
sonogram, 221, 228; defined 356
source material: *see* factor concentrate – purity
spanking: *see* discipline

specialty pharmacy, 104, 105, 106, 107, 108, 110, 112, 253; defined 356
spontaneous bleed, 26, 27
    defined, 356
    joints and, 47, 113
    prophylaxis and, 113, 117, 118, 129
    severe hemophilia and, 152
    See also breakthrough bleed, severe hemophilia
spontaneous mutation, 34
SSDI: see Social Security Disability Income
SSI: see Supplemental Security Income
strep throat, 50, 80
stretching, 187
subcutaneous, 40, 42, 55, 80, 298 ch. 13 n.10; defined 356
Supplemental Security Income (SSI), 269, 271
swelling, 170, 172
    allergic reactions and, 158
    blood tests and, 80
    compartment syndrome and, 42
    deep vein thrombosis and, 297 ch. 7 n.4
    eye bleeds and, 51
    gastrointestinal bleeds and, 51
    infusions and, 157
    joint bleeds and, 47, 48
    joint injury and, 72
    major bleeds and, 45-46, 51, 55
    pocket infection and, 123
    throat bleeds and, 45, 50-51, 80
symptomatic bleeding, 219
symptomatic carrier, 219-20, 293-94 ch. 2 n.7; defined 357
synovitis, 48 fig. 3.1; defined 357
synovium, 48 fig. 3.1, 81; defined 357

T

target joint
    defined, 357
    joint bleed and, 153, 166
    limitations and, 184, 190
    prophylaxis and, 117, 119, 120, 126
teething, 77-79, 90
tertiary prophylaxis, 117, 128, 129; defined 357; *see also* prophylaxis
throat bleed, 50-51
thrombosis, 239, 297 ch. 7 n.4; defined 357; *see also* deep vein thrombosis
titer, 243; defined 357; *see also* Bethesda unit, high-titer inhibitor, low-titer inhibitor
Title V Children with Special Healthcare Needs Programs (CSHCNP), 269
tongue bleed, 79, 154
tooth, 78
    brushing, 154
    extraction, 217, 220, 235
    loss, 154
tourniquet, 40, 80, 116, 147, 202; defined 357
transfusion, 28, 331
travel
    letter, 162, 163
    planning for, 161, 162, 164, 166, 297 ch. 9 n.8, 300 ch. 17 n.2
triage nurse: *see* nurse – ER triage
TRICARE, 267
Tylenol, 81, 90, 338; *see also* acetaminophen

U

ultrapure, 95, 96, 100, 111, 112, 295 ch. 6 n.3; defined 358; *see also* factor concentrate – purity
ultrasound, 59, 221, 226, 297 ch. 7 n.4; defined 358
umbilical cord, 40, 225, 226

urinary tract (UT), 155
    bleed, 153, 154–55
UT: *see* urinary tract

V

vaccination, 37, 40, 42, 43, 55, 296 ch. 7 n.3
vaccine
    DTaP, 53
    hib, 53
    hepatitis A (HAV), 53, 329
    hepatitis B (HBV), 53
    MMR, 53
    pneumococcal, 53
    polio, 53
    varicella, 53
vacuum extraction, 223, 224, 225
VAD: *see* central venous access device
vaginal birth, 223, 224, 225; *see also* childbirth
vasoconstriction, 21, 22, 23 fig. 2.1, 35
vein, 20–21
    blood test and, 40, 43, 80
    CVAD and, 121, 122, 125
    deep vein thrombosis and, 124, 125, 297 ch. 7 n.4
    defined, 358
    femoral, 68
    immune tolerance therapy and, 240
    infusion and, 27, 28, 64, 86, 88, 116, 158
    jugular, 68; defined 350
    muscle bleed and, 46
    physical activity and, 183, 186
    prophylaxis and, 115, 122, 126, 128, 296–97 ch. 7 n.2 & 5
    umbilical, 223

venipuncture and, 61, 63
venipuncture, 28, 61, 63, 113, 116, 121, 125, 157, 297 ch. 7 n.5; defined 358
venous access device (VAD): *see* central venous access device
Veterans Health Care Act (VHCA), 296 ch. 6 n.10
VHCA: *see* Veterans Health Care Act
viral
    contamination, 199
    disease, 51, 98, 324, 328, 333 App. D n.2
    inactivation, 97, 98-99, 102, 296 ch. 6 n.6 & 7, 324, 327-333, 333 App. D n.5 & 6; defined 358
    removal, 96, 97
    transmission, 96, 111
vomiting of blood, 50, 51
von Willebrand disease (VWD), 24, 101, 293 ch. 2 n.4; defined 358
von Willebrand factor (VWF), 99, 293 ch. 2 n.4; defined 359

W
West Nile virus, 98
wheezing, 158, 294 ch. 3 n.7
withdrawal, product, 160, 332; defined 359

X
X chromosome, defined 349; *see also* chromosome
x-ray, 59, 61, 62, 65, 71, 88, 158, 294 ch. 4 n.3

Y
Y chromosome; defined, 359; *see also* chromosome

Notes